LOCKED IN

IN

LOCKED

OUT

LOCKED IN

SHAWN JENNINGS

LOCKED OUT

Surviving a Brainstem Stroke

DUNDURN
TORONTO

Publisher: Scott Fraser | Acquiring editor: Rachel Spence | Editor: Dominic Farrell
Cover designer: Laura Boyle
Printer: Webcom, a division of Marquis Book Printing Inc.

Library and Archives Canada Cataloguing in Publication

Title: Locked In Locked Out : Surviving a Brainstem Stroke / Shawn Jennings.
Names: Jennings, Shawn, author.
Description: Originally published: Saint John, N.B. : DreamCatcher Pub., 2002.
Identifiers: Canadiana (print) 20190189533 | Canadiana (ebook) 20190189541 | ISBN 9781459745995 (softcover) | ISBN 9781459746008 (PDF) | ISBN 9781459746015 (EPUB)
Subjects: LCSH: Jennings, Shawn—Health. | LCSH: Cerebrovascular disease—Patients— Biography. | LCSH: Paralytics—Patients—Biography. | LCSH: Coma—Patients—Biography. | LCSH: Physicians—Biography. | LCGFT: Autobiographies.
Classification: LCC RC388.5 .J45 2020 | DDC 362.1968/10092—dc23

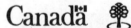

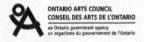
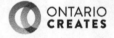

We acknowledge the support of the Canada Council for the Arts and the Ontario Arts Council for our publishing program. We also acknowledge the financial support of the Government of Ontario, through the Ontario Book Publishing Tax Credit and Ontario Creates, and the Government of Canada.

Printed and bound in Canada.

VISIT US AT

 dundurn.com |  @dundurnpress |  dundurnpress | 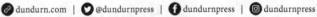 dundurnpress

Dundurn
3 Church Street, Suite 500
Toronto, Ontario, Canada
M5E 1M2

For my wife, Jill, whose love sustained me and lit my way

FOREWORD

Randy Dickinson, CM
Chairperson, Premier's Council on Disabilities

Locked in Locked Out is a compelling read. This book describes the personal journey of an adult who suddenly becomes very disabled and is forced to adapt his whole way of living. Shawn writes in a simple, heartfelt style. He manages to pique our intellectual curiosity and tug at our hearts as he tells his unvarnished truth.

Imagine that you are a very busy and popular family doctor with a large practice. You have a full life, with a loving wife, three children, and a dog. You enjoy walking in the woods and spending time outdoors at your cottage and doing chores there and around the house as a stress relief from your demanding work schedule.

You are very engaged with your patients and even do house calls for some of those who are unable to make it to the clinic or hospital for ongoing treatment. You love your job as a doctor.

Suddenly, you suffer a brainstem stroke, which leaves you paralyzed, unable to move your limbs, unable to walk, unable to speak, unable to breathe on your own, unable to swallow or eat, and unable to form facial expressions to indicate how you are feeling or what mood you are in. You are locked in.

This is the story of Dr. Shawn Jennings.

As a long-time disability advocate and a person who lives with a disability myself, I have read countless books and articles on the subject of disability and how people have reacted to their situation. Dr. Jennings has managed to put together a detailed and very personal description of his road to recovery, how he coped day by day with the dramatic adjustment in his personal situation, and how he has been able to function with his reality, going forward. He is also able, as he is a medically trained doctor, to convey exactly what happened to him physiologically and offer insight into the nature and purpose of the medical treatment that he received and rehabilitation process he underwent.

Reading this book, you become engrossed in Shawn's reaction to the situation he finds himself in. He conveys so well his frustration about being unable to speak or even demonstrate his emotions through facial expressions, and the anguish he suffers because he is unable to communicate when he is in pain or being tormented by a housefly crawling on his face. All of the incredible difficulties associated with being locked in are shared here.

Shawn gives significant credit to the unconditional love and ongoing support of his wife, Jill, and the help of the rest of his family members as he struggled with the challenge of coping with his disability. Jill had worked with Shawn as the manager of his medical practice and was also a nurse herself. Perhaps this prepared her somewhat for being able to assume the role of caregiver and emotional bedrock for Shawn as he tried to deal with the transition from respected family doctor to a highly dependent patient learning to accommodate a serious disability.

In a certain way, this book is partially a love story; it is clear that this couple share an unconditional love that would not be suppressed by the physical changes Shawn experienced. Unfortunately, when a person becomes seriously disabled and requires significant support, it is not uncommon for couples to separate and divorce because of the stress and challenges that such a disability can create. I am happy to report that this was not the case with Jill and Shawn Jennings.

Shortly after receiving immediate medical intervention at the local hospital in Saint John, Shawn was transferred to a rehabilitation centre in Fredericton known as the Stan Cassidy Centre for Rehabilitation. This was where Shawn began the long and difficult journey to restoring, as much as possible, his ability to function. This was where the road to a life with a semblance of independence began.

Readers will be intrigued to follow the detailed synopsis of the rehabilitation program that Shawn went through to restore his ability to swallow and eat, to breathe unassisted, to communicate with others, and to regain some level of physical control over his body that would enable him to be more self-sufficient and to use a power wheelchair for mobility.

Shawn describes clearly the various interventions and therapies that were used in his rehabilitation and the moments of frustration and satisfaction he experienced during that process. Progress was slow and achieved only with a lot of hard work and effort on his part — and, as Shawn makes a point of noting, the help of his knowledgeable and compassionate therapists.

Locked In Locked Out is not only an outstanding description of a patient's medical journey as he tries to recover from a brainstem stroke, but also a wonderful portrait of an ordinary man. In the book, we see Shawn's intelligence, his insight into the people around him, his humanity, his love for his wife and family, and his outstanding sense of humour. Shawn really enjoys a laugh and is not at all averse to laughing at himself. I can vividly remember his hearty, rip-snorting laugh.

Given the fact that, because of his condition, Shawn was forced to live inside his head to an unusual degree, it is not surprising that the book includes meditation and introspection. Shawn offers his thoughts on spirituality and on how bodily injuries can affect the inner person. Although he is frank about his own feelings, Shawn never tries to persuade readers that his own observations and conclusions are the right ones; he is not someone who is interested in interfering with the spiritual beliefs of others.

I had the pleasure of working with Shawn for the many years that he served as an active board member of the Premier's Council on Disabilities and with the New Brunswick Health Council. Shawn was also affiliated with Dalhousie Medical School and was a member of a national committee of physicians living with a disability, and he made a huge difference to their deliberations. He also helped lobby for a modern version of the Stan Cassidy Centre for Rehabilitation, which was built and opened in 2006.

I am very honoured to be asked by Shawn to write this fore-word, and I consider myself very lucky to know him and to be able to call Shawn and Jill Jennings our friends.

Enjoy the book!

INTRODUCTION

If a person's brainstem, which is the transit area between the brain and the spinal cord, is damaged, the results can be quite devastating. Both sides of the body can be paralyzed, and speech, swallowing, and involuntary functions such as breathing can be affected. A cerebral stroke, a common type of stroke, damages one side of the brain and one side of the body and may affect speech and swallowing. A cerebral stroke often hinders the thinking processes of the brain, resulting in problems with finding the right words, personality changes, impaired memory, and a myriad of other processing problems in the brain. A brainstem stroke does not damage the brain, but leaves a cognitively normal person imprisoned inside a body with no movement. I found myself in this condition — aptly called "locked-in syndrome" — in May of 1999, at the age of forty-five.

Some people, early in my rehabilitation, mentioned that I should write a book about my experiences of being locked in. At first I gave it little thought, but the idea had been planted.

Eventually, the book became a way for my brain to focus when all I could do was think (which was driving me crazy). I wrote it in my mind, not knowing if I would ever be able to physically write.

But why would anyone want to read my memoir? I felt so alone when I was locked in. It would have been comforting to hear from other brainstem stroke survivors about their experiences. I later found books on the subject, written by other survivors, but in one the survivor dies and in another the survivor has a second stroke. Perhaps I could write a book for my fellow stroke survivors that was more uplifting and hopeful.

If I was going to write a book for brainstem stroke survivors, I decided, I needed to be sincere and honest, even at the risk of embarrassing myself. I would never have publicly divulged such personal thoughts and details in a memoir without the focus of being sincere with my fellow survivors. I hope this book will be of some small comfort to a new survivor somewhere, sometime. If this book achieves that, then I will be happy.

But brainstem stroke survivors would be an extremely small target audience to write for, no matter how valuable the book was to them. I also needed to make the book interesting to average readers. Perhaps those readers would find it interesting to hear a doctor's perspective on suddenly becoming a very dependent patient or to read about someone's reaction to being locked inside a non-functioning body. I have included many stories about my patients throughout the book because these memories either gave me perspective in my time of hardship or taught me invaluable life lessons. Perhaps, I thought, mixing my narrative with these tales would pique the interest of those average readers.

I have tried to speak like a patient and not a doctor, but that may have been impossible at times, and for that I'm sorry.

I started typing with one finger, once I could move my left hand, so the actual writing of this book became a therapeutic secondary gain. I began during Christmas of 1999 and finished around Christmas of 2001.

I didn't know much about publishing, nor did I have any expectation that a publishing company would want to publish the book, so I jumped at the chance when a local company, DreamCatcher Publishing, said they were interested. I initially thought a few local people who knew or had heard of me might want to read my memoir, but I never expected the number or variety of people who eventually read *Locked In Locked Out*.

Locked In Locked Out was first published in 2002, and since then many people have suggested that I write an update. I couldn't imagine why I would: I didn't have enough to say to warrant a whole new edition. I had no intention of revisiting *Locked In Locked Out*, and I hadn't read a page of my memoir in eighteen years.

I submitted my third book, *A Forgivable Indecision,* digitally to a few publishers across Canada in 2018, and to my surprise Dundurn Press said they would be interested in publishing a new edition of my memoir if I'd revise it and add updates. I thought it might be a compelling project for me, so I agreed.

I revised a lot of the first-edition material. I hope I've improved the grammar and sentence structure. I've added a new patient story and chapters of new material at the end to update my life for readers. I've chosen to remove all the names of the physicians who cared for me. The first names of my patients and other health care professionals may or may not be correct; I intentionally did this to protect their privacy.

I could not have lived through the ordeal of being locked in without the love and caring of my wife. It was she who stayed by my side from day one. It was she I cried with. It was she who wiped my nose and suctioned out my trachea, yet gently wiped my brow. It was she who lifted my spirits with a simple smile, yet it was she who cajoled me into trying harder during my long months of rehabilitation. It was her love that made me realize what life is all about. It was her love that sustained me throughout this crisis. This book is a small product of that love. I love you, Jill, and this book is dedicated to you.

CHAPTER 1
THE EVENT

May 13, 1999, was bright and promising, or so I thought. The smell of new grass was in the air. It was the type of day you waited for all winter. I got up and had a shower, not knowing that it would be the last time I would have a shower for months. I packed my golf clothes in my sports bag and headed downstairs. I ate my regular cereal while I marvelled at the glorious day that awaited me. I talked to Jenny, my dog, and then climbed into my truck without a care — and without a thought about what I would soon consider a dream: the ability to drive. Soon I was heading down the highway for the hospital.

I was a family physician who had been in practice for twenty years. I enjoyed my life. I took pleasure in the patient-doctor interaction and liked the variety of complaints that a family physician sees. The one thing I never enjoyed was the constant time stress inherent in this work. There was always the need to balance giving enough time to each patient and seeing everyone who wanted to be seen. But after twenty years, I think I had moulded my practice to fit my personality.

This was to be a special day: I was taking the afternoon off for a golf game. An afternoon with no phone calls, no thinking about diagnoses, no questions to answer; nothing but easy banter with my buddies and a nice walk on a pleasant day. The golf itself was secondary to the social interaction and the surroundings.

With this on my mind, I headed into the hospital. I made my rounds without incident. All of my patients were doing as expected. One of the last patients I saw was Pauli, a lady in her early sixties who had scleroderma, a progressive disease that would soon enter the terminal stages for her. Scleroderma is caused when too much collagen is laid down in the tissues of the affected body part, which causes a fibrosis, or stiffness. The skin loses its elasticity and normal cells are displaced. The cause for this excess collagen is unknown.

She had been well, looking younger than her age, until about five years before, when this insidious disease started. It had progressed at an alarming rate. At first it caused the skin on her hands to tighten. Her fingers were unable to bend and the skin had split open over her knuckles, leaving open sores that wouldn't heal. Then the skin around her mouth tightened, causing a loss of expression and difficulty with speech. Her legs became involved, making walking impossible. Next the disease started to work its way into her digestive system, stealing her ability to swallow or digest food, and she had chronic diarrhea. The week before, we'd had to insert a gastrostomy tube into her stomach, bypassing her mouth and esophagus, to give her nutrition in the form of a liquid supplement. I had been torn by this decision, as the supplement would prolong the inevitable. I was sure that what life remained to her would be of poor quality, filled with pain and suffering, but she had made my decision easier with her wish to keep going. Finally, in what I believed was going to be the final straw, the disease had started to affect her kidneys.

To complicate things further, she had experienced a stroke when the disease had spread to her blood vessels. In addition to paralysis, the stroke had caused aphasia, or damage to the areas of the brain involved with language, hampering her ability to communicate verbally.

Her family had been very supportive. Her husband had kept her at home as long as he could until the diarrhea, immobility, and other factors led us to admit her to hospital. When I went to see her that day, she had just been moved from an active ward to this chronic care ward. She would be the last patient I would see.

"Good morning, Pauli," I said.

"Aaaa," she responded as best she could.

"Did you have a good night?"

"Mmmmm, Au ha soo diaea," she tried to say.

"Some diarrhea?" I guessed.

"Aaaa."

"Did you take the MCT oil with your meal last night?" MCT oil is a substitute for butter or margarine that is easy to digest.

"Ugh!" She grimaced.

"Well, I'll have to look at your chart to see if there are any meds that maybe we should look at. What did they give you to eat last night?" As soon as I said it, I knew this was a foolish question. How could she respond? "Sorry!" I said sheepishly.

She chuckled.

"I'll ask the nurse." I proceeded to examine her hands, which were grossly contracted, like a bird's claw, and just as delicate. Her mouth was drawn back, exposing her upper teeth, but she could still smile, as she was doing now. I carefully lifted up her pyjama top so I could see her gastrostomy tube. It looked to be healing just fine, despite the scleroderma.

"Be good!" I said. She nodded, and I strolled away to examine her chart. After I had written my progress notes and typed my orders into the computer, I left the floor. I left the hospital quite quickly and jumped into my truck. Rolling down the windows, I breathed in the fresh air — no air conditioning for me today. As I neared my office, I looked out at the clear blue sea beyond the harbour and once again marvelled at the day. Just the morning to get through and I would be free. I drove into the parking lot at my clinic and turned my head to back up. It was approximately 9:00 a.m.

As I turned my head, a peculiar sensation hit me: my vision started to move backward and forward. My ears began to ring. *Vertigo!* I thought. The McDonald's sign across the street shifted back and forth. I noticed a man sitting in his car beside me. *Hope I don't make a fool of myself!*

I was due to start in the office now. I felt I couldn't walk, so I called my wife, who worked as a nurse in my office. I was lucky she was there, because she usually didn't work on Thursdays. She later told me that I was doubly lucky, as there was no battery life left on my cellphone after that call.

My receptionist answered the phone and I asked to speak to Jill. "I won't be able to make it in," I said. "I'm awful dizzy!"

"Where are you?" Jill said, alarmed at the concern in my voice.

"In the upper parking lot."

I don't remember much about the next few minutes until I saw Jill in front of my truck. She found the door open and my seat belt unfastened. I don't remember doing this, but I vaguely recall feeling hot, so I may have opened the door for air.

I again told her that I was dizzy. She felt that I should go to the hospital and helped me out of the truck. I staggered over to the back seat of her car, which I had happened to park beside. Having great difficulty arranging myself into a comfortable position, I thought this was a really strong attack of vertigo.

Jill drove around to the other side of the building to tell my receptionist and my patients, who had already arrived, what we were doing. While she was gone, I realized I was going in and out of consciousness. I also started to think that this was more than vertigo. My right hand was feeling heavy and numb. I became aware that my breathing was laboured. My lips were pouting and I could almost hear myself snore. I felt I should stop this, straighten up, but weariness overcame me. Sleep would feel so good.

Jill was gone but seconds. When she returned, she was alarmed at my condition. I could hear her asking me questions. I wanted to respond, to tell her about my hand, to tell her what I suspected was happening to me, but when I tried to speak, all that came out was a garbled "mmmm." As she drove to the hospital, I became more unconscious. As if in a dream, I could hear her imploring me to keep talking and stay awake. My only response was a deep groan or a snore.

My final moment of awareness was in front of the emergency department. I saw and felt a male nurse and an orderly, both of whom I knew, lift me out of the car. I heard someone say, "We just saw him this morning!" That was the last thing I heard as I lapsed into the sleep I seemed to need so desperately.

CHAPTER 2
THE DIAGNOSIS

I was in deep, deep trouble, and I was the only one who knew it. I was having a stroke and I couldn't tell them — I was in a coma. After examinations and blood tests, the emergency room (ER) staff had ruled out the most common causes of sudden loss of consciousness and sent me for a CT scan. Unfortunately, it was read as negative, not through an error in judgment but because of poor quality. My deep breathing, with a raucous snore, caused my head to move, so they could not get a clear picture. However, even if the picture had been perfect, it's possible that the diagnosis might have eluded them at this point.

More time was spent waiting for some clinical change that might indicate what was going on. As it turned out, this was time I could ill afford. The ER doctor was perplexed. Based on the results of the CT scan, it appeared that no major event had occurred in my brain to cause this sudden loss of consciousness. At first, the doctor was relieved that the CT scan showed no tumour or blood in my brain. He entertained the possibility that I had had a seizure and I was now in a postictal, or post-seizure, state. He was waiting for me to awaken, but I remained unconscious.

My wife was becoming frantic. When she was told there was a lot of distortion on the first CT scan, she implored the staff to do another because she knew I hadn't had a seizure. They eventually sent me for another scan, but I had to be returned to the ER because my breathing was even worse. Another scan would have been a waste of time. They recommended intubation.

About this time, the neurologist who was on call that day examined me and was concerned I was locked in, totally paralyzed from head to toe and unable to communicate.

To intubate a patient, a medication is first given to paralyze the muscles. Then a hollow tube with a balloon on one end is inserted down the patient's throat and into the larynx, or windpipe. Some people's anatomy makes this hard to do. I was one of these people. After a few failed attempts by the ER doctors, an anesthetist had to be called down to try the intubation. I later ended up with aspiration pneumonia because of these many failed attempts. Aspiration pneumonia can occur when oral secretions, ladened with bacteria, pass into the lungs. Coughing normally prevents this, but in a patient who is unconscious, this defensive mechanism is absent, so the oral secretions may settle into the lungs undisturbed.

The staff were now breathing for me by pumping a bag attached to my intubation tube. I was sent back for another CT scan. This time, something was seen. I appeared to have a clot in my left vertebral artery, a major artery in the neck. No blood was flowing to my brainstem. I was having a brainstem stroke.

A stroke usually happens when a clot interrupts normal blood flow. The clot forms in a blood vessel that has been narrowed by cholesterol plaque. It then either blocks the vessel at this point or flies off and blocks another smaller vessel some distance away.

This same scenario happens in heart attacks. In fact, both strokes and heart attacks are called *infarcts*, and some medical professionals refer to strokes as brain attacks.

Blood carries oxygen to the body's cells, and without oxygen they quickly die. In a stroke, time is critical. As more time passes after the stroke starts, more cells die and more damage is done. It was now after 12:00 p.m. and my stroke had started at 9:00 a.m.

The brainstem looks after very primitive functions such as sleeping, eating, breathing, and controlling heart rate — functions necessary for even the lowest of creatures in the evolutionary chain. Also, all the commands from the brain to the rest of the body pass through this narrow canal. A stroke in this area usually causes paralysis to both sides of the body. The patient can't breathe properly, can't swallow or speak, and often has double vision. Only the eyelids are able to move. Most people who have a brainstem stroke don't survive. Those who do are significantly impaired. A few stay locked in; that is, their brain is functioning normally but they are unable to move, swallow, or talk. Most survivors of a brainstem stroke go through a locked-in phase and then improve.

As I revise this memoir twenty years after my stroke, treatment and early recognition of brainstem strokes continue to improve. Emergency physicians have learned to be aware when a person with a history of neck pain is brought into the ER in a comatose state so that they can rule out a brainstem stroke. The technology of detection and treatment of strokes has also advanced in the past twenty years.

In my case, some damage to the brainstem must have already occurred. To leave me would probably have meant death. Radiologists attempted a cerebral angiography to dissolve the clot with medication. This procedure involves making an incision in the groin and manipulating a small tube up the femoral artery (the main artery in the thigh) to the aorta and then up to the vertebral artery in the back of the neck. After a few failed attempts, they asked an interventional cardiologist to help.

Together they again attempted the procedure but ran into problems: my left vertebral artery seemed to be narrower than expected and it started to bleed outside the vessel wall when they injected the clot-busting drug. They realized then that the clot had formed from a tear in the artery, and dissolving this patchwork was letting blood pass through the inner vessel wall.

Now they had a real problem. If they continued the drug, I would die. To leave me and do nothing would mean more cells would die from lack of oxygen.

By judicial use of the clot-busting drug and physical manipulation, they created enough of a canal to let some blood trickle through. The problem now was to maintain this flow and prevent further clotting.

They decided to use heparin, which is a drug used to prevent clots and dissolve them, although in a much slower fashion than other clot-busting drugs. Heparin was slowly infused through an intravenous line in my arm, with caution because it, too, could cause the artery to bleed more, but my chances were better with heparin than without. In this precarious state, I was sent to the neurological intensive care unit (NICU) under the care of a neurologist. I am indebted to all the health care professionals involved for saving my life.

Meanwhile, the head of the radiology department had taken my wife to his office to explain the diagnosis and angiography. He let her stay in his office for the afternoon. My mother, Doreen McLaughlin, joined her at this point. When he returned some time later, he didn't have good news. He thought Jill should probably call in my children to see me.

CHAPTER 3
THE CAUSE

Two weeks prior to this stroke, I had almost been involved in an automobile collision. I had just finished some minor surgery at St. Joseph's Hospital and was heading to the Saint John Regional Hospital, also known as the Regional. As I entered an intersection, a blue Ford F-150 driving in the opposite direction turned in front of me. I was about to hit it broadside. I had never been in an automobile accident, but I was sure this was it. There was a girl in the front passenger seat and our eyes met. I thought I was about to slam into her. As I prayed *Dear God, no!*, I slammed on the brakes. The driver, oblivious to the danger, never altered her speed. I came to a screeching halt, mere inches from the pickup.

It is strange the things you observe in a crisis. I clearly remember a man in a vehicle to my right shaking his head at the near collision.

Later that morning, I felt a vague ache in my neck while making rounds at the hospital. At noon, I was having lunch with a friend of mine when I experienced a strange warm sensation in my neck and felt off balance. I grabbed the edge of the table to keep steady and didn't say anything to my companion. I expect that was the moment my blood vessel started to bleed. As I left the lunch, I felt a little wobbly on my feet but thought nothing of it.

The ache intensified that afternoon in the office. I thought I had a whiplash. I have treated many patients with this malady over the years, so it was kind of interesting to me to actually experience it. Some whiplash injuries can become chronic, but most are minor and get better with time. I was sure mine would prove to be mild. I took an anti-inflammatory medication and finished up my day.

Later that night and throughout the week, I took anti-inflammatories and occasionally put wet heat on my neck. I was not concerned. I continued to run my office, oversee my patients in hospital, and do my chores at home. My first golf game of the season was coming up and I thought the exercise might actually do my neck some good.

Patients who have the best outcomes with whiplash are those who can ignore the pain and continue their normal activities. For some people, the pain is too intense to ignore and they start to fear bending their neck, and as a result they end up with a chronic, stiff, painful condition. I was determined not to be one of those.

It was about a week after my whiplash that my golf partner and I decided to tee off. My first hole of the year was a success: I had a par and hit the ball well. It would be the last hole I played well, ever.

As I bent over to retrieve my ball from the hole, I felt odd. I walked over to the second tee and started to feel dizzy. My legs felt weak, rubbery. *That's funny*, I thought. Although I had eaten my lunch, I felt somewhat hypoglycemic, as if my blood sugar was low.

Somehow, I hit a perfect drive down the middle of the fairway. My friend hit one into the rough. What was his excuse! We chatted as we walked up the fairway, but I was feeling very shaky. I hadn't told him how I felt.

He left me to find his ball. I prayed he would find it easily, because I didn't think I could walk over to where he was. He found the ball and hit it. As I stood over my ball, my legs felt even weaker. I was dizzy and nauseated, and my mouth was dry. I hit the ball more from muscle memory than from skill and landed it just off the green.

I putted quickly in two strokes, not really caring about the outcome. On our way to the third hole, we walked down a little hill. I really wasn't sure if I would make it.

"I'm feeling a bit woozy," I said as I sat down on a bench. "I'm dizzy, sort of weak in the knees. Everything's going around. You go ahead and hit."

He drove the ball up to an elevated green. It was now my turn, but I knew I couldn't continue. "I can't do it," I said. "I don't think I can even walk back."

I noticed a group approaching behind us with an electric golf car. When they reached us, I asked if one of them wouldn't mind driving me back to my car.

I clambered onto the golf car, holding my golf clubs precariously against my body, and we headed off. I was afraid I might vomit as the bumping and to-and-fro motion of the golf car sent my head spinning. Back at my truck, I somehow managed to get my clubs into the back. After the golf car ride, my head was really spinning and I had great difficulty staying on my feet. Holding on to the truck, I made my way into the passenger seat. I felt very weak and broke out into a sweat. I couldn't focus on my surroundings. I sat there, waiting for my friend.

When he came, we decided to head to the emergency department, which was just down the road. I felt like a fool walking into emergency with my golf shoes on and my friend supporting me. After the nurses took the routine measurements, blood draws, and history, the same ER doctor who would see me the day of my stroke a week later came in. He took a history and examined me, finding fluid in my middle ear.

"Seems as though you have vertigo, probably caused by that fluid in your middle ear," he said. "I'm going to set you up with an IV and give you metoclopramide. Okay?"

I mentioned my whiplash injury. He and I couldn't fathom how that type of injury could give me these symptoms, so I agreed to his plan. But something was bothering me: I often have fluid in my middle ears. I have allergic rhinitis, or hay fever, which can block my Eustachian, or auditory tubes. It has been a chronic problem since I was a youngster, but it had never caused vertigo before. I maintained my nonchalant demeanour and accepted the verdict without showing my apprehension. I was the macho doctor.

After I had spent some time lying on the stretcher and had received the IV metoclopramide, the vertigo started to subside. My wife arrived and soon I was well enough to go home. As we walked out, I noted that my gait was wider, but this wasn't unusual considering the fact I had just had a bout of vertigo.

An otolaryngologist — an ear, nose, and throat surgeon — who was a partner at my medical clinic agreed to see me the next day. He lanced my tympanic membrane, or eardrum, and drained the excess fluid from my middle ear.

This procedure was done on Friday, and that weekend I lay low. A patient phoned me at home on Friday afternoon, complaining of severe pain in her leg. She had diabetes and I feared her artery might have suddenly become blocked. I was in no condition to see her and told her to go immediately to the ER. I hated not being available for her in her time of need, but it had to be. It turned out that the artery was blocked; she would lose the leg.

That weekend, I continued to apply heat to my aching neck and took an occasional anti-inflammatory. My gait remained unsteady, but not remarkably so. I felt like I could work on Monday. At the hospital, while I was seeing my patients, I happened to meet a neurologist, who would later be involved on the day of my stroke, and I told him my tale. I was not convinced that my ears had caused the vertigo. He had a few minutes, so he took me to an exam room in the hospital.

During his exam, I was surprised to find that I absolutely could not walk heel to toe. He felt things were not normal and given my vertigo, gait disturbance, and pain, I warranted a CT scan. He said his secretary would call me when that was booked. I expected to have to wait a week or two for the scan, but I felt better knowing further investigation was coming.

The stroke happened three days later. I have often wondered if the results would have been different if I had voiced my concerns more in the ER the week before. I didn't believe the fluid had caused the vertigo. Did the fact that I was a physician being evaluated by a colleague prevent me from questioning his judgment? What if the CT scan had been done when I saw the neurologist three days before the stroke? But I didn't think it was an emergency; I was walking around the hospital, making rounds. What if the problem had been detected on the first CT scan I had in the ER during my stroke?

What-ifs. When something bad like this happens, there are always a lot of what-ifs. Some people get hung up on them. I found out early that you can "what if?" all you like, but it won't change anything. Bad things happen. Accept them and move on.

In the NICU on Thursday evening, I awoke from my coma. My first conscious thought was *My God, they've put a catheter in my dink! This is serious!*

CHAPTER 4
THE NEUROLOGICAL
INTENSIVE CARE UNIT

When I awoke, I was aware of nurses hovering around me. I wanted to speak to them, but I found myself unable to. *No wonder. They've put a tube in my throat.* I slowly became aware that I was intubated and a respirator was breathing for me.

It did not concern me that I had been intubated. I was strangely comfortable with my situation. It was not long before the neurologist appeared. He explained that I had had a stroke and asked me if I understood. He told me to blink once for yes and twice for no. I blinked once. He then asked me simple questions, to which I responded appropriately. He told the nurses I was thinking clearly. I thought, *Of course I'm okay; I've had a little mini stroke. Come on, guys!*

Jill arrived at my side soon thereafter. She stroked my hair and patted my hand. The closeness and love I felt for this woman at that moment mingled with the warmth that lingered from my comatose state.

I had no near-death experience that I can remember. But despite all that had been done — the traumatic intubation, the angiogram, the catheterization, and the IVs — I awoke feeling great. I felt as though I had just had a good sleep, or something good had just happened. I really didn't want to wake up. Had I experienced something? Was this just a normal physiological response after a coma? I don't know, but I'll never be afraid of a coma in the future.

I was not at all concerned about what had befallen me. It didn't seem important. It was like waking up in your grandma's home wrapped in a toasty blanket, or on a foggy morning when you have nothing to get up for, so you can curl up for a longer snooze. The respirator pushing air into my lungs, my inability to move, the IVs — all of these things that should have panicked me had no effect. I was calm.

Later in my rehabilitation, I comforted a mourning mother. Her son, eighteen years of age, had had a congenital heart condition that had run its course, and he had undergone a heart transplant. Unfortunately, the new heart failed, and he lived for a number of days without a heart until a second heart was found. The second transplant was successful, but the days of trying to keep him alive on the heart bypass machine took their toll and he hemorrhaged. Unbeknownst to me, the mother was afraid he had suffered while he was comatose without a heart. I happened to mention to her that while I was in my coma, I had felt very restful. I have no idea why I even mentioned this. The mother was shocked and started to cry. She softly thanked me for giving her such a beautiful gift.

As a doctor, I used to tell grieving or worried relatives that their loved ones in a coma were not suffering. I said it to comfort them, but truthfully, although I thought it was probably true, I didn't know for certain. Now I can say with conviction that they are not suffering. If you have a loved one with cancer or any terminal illness who is going in and out of consciousness, they are not suffering. A coma is a restful state of mind. Welcome it.

My memories of the next few hours and through the night are hazy. I remember seeing my children that evening — or do I? I was restless that night, wanting to shift my body, but it wouldn't respond. Next morning, the neurologist told me they were going to do another angiogram. This news elicited no fear or anxiety in me. I met it with that same unconcerned attitude I felt about my whole situation. I must have been in a semi-comatose state because I remember only moments of the trip down. The only part of the procedure I remember is my colleagues squealing, "We got it! It's gone!"

What they were saying is that the clot in my artery had dissolved overnight from the use of heparin. I would live, but in what condition? No one could say for sure at this point, but the neurologist took my family aside and explained to them what they could expect based on the damage shown on CT scan.

"Your dad is probably going to live, but there has been a lot of damage," he said. "His brain function will be fine. He knows you, and his personality will be the same as it always was. He won't be able to speak, but I think he can retrain his speech to a certain extent. I don't know how much he will get back in his arms and legs, but he probably won't walk. The injury affected his swallowing, so we will have to perform a tracheotomy. Hopefully, in time, he will learn to swallow and the breathing tube can come out. In the meantime, he will need tube feedings."

The neurologist's assessment would prove to be quite accurate. My wife and kids later told me that they had no questions for him. They were trying to get used to the idea that I was critically ill. Their world had suddenly changed, yet there were no distinguishing features to mark today from yesterday. Everybody, sooner or later, experiences events that change their life forever. My event had occurred.

Over the course of the next few days, my circumstance became more apparent to me: I'd had a stroke but a most unusual one: a brainstem stroke. I searched my memory, trying to recall if I had ever seen one in my practice. No, in twenty years I had never come across this condition. I thought it couldn't be too bad. After all, I could feel. I could feel my toes, hands, face, everything. I seemed to have no sensory deficit.

In some ways, I would have welcomed a loss of sensation. My limbs rebelled at not being able to move. I ached in different areas of my body. The nurses turned me every two hours. It was a relief from my agony, but a few minutes later, the pain would start in some other area of my body. I was unable to scream out or make any commotion to signal to anyone, so I had to wait until someone happened to come by. Then I would try to make my distress apparent by batting my eyelashes furiously. An anatomy lesson would then take place.

"Is something the matter, Shawn?"

One blink.

"Are you in pain?"

One blink.

"Is it your arm?"

Two blinks.

"Your head?"

Two blinks.

"Your legs?"

One blink.

"Is it your right leg?"

One blink.

"Is it your calf?"

One blink.

The nurse would rectify the problem, which usually meant just placing the aching body part in a different position. Sometimes there was more than one pain, and I soon learned that trying to communicate about multiple areas of my body only caused confusion. I decided that I had to indicate which area hurt the most and then be content with some relief.

The worst time was the night. Nurses don't want to disturb a patient's sleep time, so they come around only on schedule. I spent many hours trying novel ways to ignore the pain. A few times, I was sure the nurses were ignoring me on purpose. I stupidly imagined that they were taking revenge upon me. For insomniacs, nighttime can create outlandish thinking, and I was not immune. As the hours passed, I monitored which area was now aching more. I would try to will the nurse to come. I thought maybe I could master telepathy. I never could.

Pain was a consistent partner for those first few weeks. Most of the time, I was unable to explain to anyone that I was in constant pain. No one saw I was in pain because I was unable to create any expression on my face. A painkiller would have been appreciated, but then the problem would have been how to monitor my recovery. With any brain injury, it's important to be able to assess how alert the patient is.

My heart broke if I waited hours for someone to come and then they didn't look at my face or understand my blinking. It was my first lesson in frustration — with many more to come. The faces of the nurses were my link to socialization. Instead of talking, I looked at them and listened to their stories. I delighted in those who chose to tell me about their lives: what their children were doing, what their husbands had done on the weekend, what repairs their cars needed. Any topic, I didn't care. It was an escape from thinking. For that is all you can do while locked in: think.

Faces, smiles — they meant so much. I will never forget my nurses, their faces, during those first few days. I felt especially close to one nurse, who had the kindest smile. She had long brown hair, often tied back. She was about my age, midforties, and had a penchant for wearing bobby socks over her white nylons. I felt like she cared, like this was more than just a job. She amused me and liked to sing while she worked around me. Her cheery attitude was what I needed. Because of my allergies, my nose is constantly congested. I usually use an allergy nasal spray at night, but this information had not been passed on to the nurses. My congested nose caused me aggravating discomfort. My inability to blow my nose would be an irritation for more than a year. This nurse recognized that the congestion was causing me problems and she used suction to clear my nasal passages. Kind of embarrassing, but such relief! Her care for me was so gentle and giving; she is always in my memory.

Music played in my head for the first few days. It was loud and classical. At first, I thought the fellow in the bed beside me was playing music awfully loud. I searched the faces of my nurses for a hint of their reaction to it. How could they let music play so loudly in an intensive care area? It was getting to be too much! *It's the middle of the night and they still allow him to play the radio! I can't sleep! Doesn't anyone care?*

It became apparent to me, sometime that night, that no one else could hear the music. It faded when someone spoke, but it was usually present. I'm not sure when I became aware of these melodies because the first night is hazy in my memory, but for sure I heard them the day after my stroke. The music was intricate but repetitive. When one song finished, it would start again — so much so that I got annoyed. I was afraid I wouldn't get rid of this phenomenon. Thankfully, after a while the melody would change.

I heard orchestration with a predominance of violins. I marvelled at how my brain could come up with such complex compositions. Although I guessed this was a side effect of my stroke,

I had never heard of this happening. None of my patients had reported this side effect. I didn't remember reading about it. I supposed that a minor clot had hit the music centre of my brain — wherever that is located — and excited it. It stopped after a few days.

A few months later, I started to wonder about the music. Why was it classical? If the music centre of my brain had been triggered, it should have generated rock, folk, or guitar music, not classical. I never listened to classical music. It was not that I hated it; I just hadn't found the time to explore it. So how could I come up with such complex compositions if I hadn't been listening to classical music? Can our brains compose this music on their own? Is it a phenomenon that occurs when a brain suddenly has no stimuli? Are we all potentially Mozart?

Could it have been heavenly music?

I have not told many people about this phenomenon because of the reactions of those I have told. Most people have become very uncomfortable when I've mentioned the music. I suppose they feel awkward because they don't know what to say.

I really don't know what I heard. Does it have a scientific explanation or was it spiritual? It has made me more attentive to the classics. I have always been somewhat spiritual, and the music I heard has only reinforced my hopes. Is there some basis of experience to the folklore of angels playing music after you die? Bugs Bunny often had a little cherub or bird playing music over his head when he got stunned.

So, there was pain, there was music, and there were tubes. There were so many tubes sticking out of my body, maybe I was supplying the music myself! If only I knew how to play them. There was the catheter in my penis, the endotracheal tube used for breathing, an arterial line, an intravenous line (maybe a couple of those), and, finally, a tube connected to pressure stockings on my legs.

I entertained myself by counting the respirator sounds. Hour after hour, the *shhhz-pop* of the respirator forced itself into my unconscious thought. When I thought I had breathed in enough air, in would come a little bit more. I never thought I was in danger or that my survival depended on the respirator, but it probably did.

The brainstem is the site of the respiratory centre. It tells the body when to inhale and exhale. Breathing is an involuntary action. We don't have to think about it for it to happen. We can override this action by using our thoughts to hold our breath. But as soon as we lose consciousness, our brainstem takes over and we start to breathe again. No one knew if my respiratory centre was damaged or not, but they couldn't take the chance, so they put me on the respirator. Then they slowly withdrew my ventilation support over a few days until I breathed on my own. I was anxious to have it removed; I felt that I could breathe without it. The respiratory therapist would come in and tell me I was doing fine, but I thought he wasn't taking any action to wean me off. Of course, he was. The respirator needed to be withdrawn slowly.

I counted as I breathed in and compared it with my last count. Other people who have been on a respirator have told me they felt like they were in a constant state of panic. I did not feel like that. The respirator sound was kind of comforting, like a grandfather clock ticking in the hall. My inability to breathe on my own did not cause me to feel like I was suffocating. I just relaxed and went with it. I tried not to fight it, nor did I feel any need to do so.

When I tired of that count, there were my pressure stockings. A pneumatic device on the floor automatically inflated them with air, and when they reached a certain pressure, a valve was released to deflate them. This kept the blood flowing through the veins in my legs to prevent clots and a condition called deep vein thrombophlebitis. If left untreated, a blood clot can break off and rush to the lungs, a life-threatening condition called a pulmonary embolism.

I counted thirty-five on, thirty-five off. I observed how close my count was each time, wondering if it was really thirty seconds or if my counting was off. Amusing little games! Although the counting drove me crazy, these little games were probably a defensive mechanism, a way to escape from my thoughts.

Living inside a dead body — what does one do? It would be a great premise for a Stephen King novel, for it was a living hell. What can one do but think? That was all I could do, and I did it constantly. I thought about my present circumstances, my life, the afterlife, my family, and my past. I didn't dwell too much on the future at first because, as I have said, I was in denial. I'd be well in a few months. However, I couldn't stop the negative thoughts from entering my mind. *What if I stay like this?*

CHAPTER 5
FURTHER THOUGHTS
IN THE NICU

I soon decided that I couldn't live day after day deep in my thoughts. I needed an escape. Ordinarily, escape for me would be reading, playing my guitar, or even work, but those weren't options now. I decided I needed a make-believe life, a place I could spend time in, maybe lead another life. Was it possible? I would later read *The Diving Bell and the Butterfly*, Jean-Dominique Bauby's account of his life as a locked-in patient after he had a brainstem stroke. He was able to let his imagination drift to places in the world he had visited in his life or read about, and he spent whole days wandering the streets of these towns fabricated in his mind. When he got tube feedings, he imagined dining on gourmet meals at fine restaurants. He could actually taste the soup, followed by lamb, lobster, or whatever. I admire his ability to transcend the present and exist in another world of his creation. I was not so strong.

I thought, *I will create a world of little creatures that live under trees and go on adventures. Ah, didn't Tolkien already do this? No matter, no one else knows. No copyrights in this world!* I set the scene, created the characters (with, of course, myself as the hero), and —

Some nurse described the cheesecake she had for lunch and I listened in.

No matter, back I went into my dream world and —

"My daughter wants these designer jeans that cost seventy-five dollars," a nurse exclaimed out of nowhere, "when she could buy a perfectly good pair, the same thing without a fancy label, for thirty dollars!"

It was impossible! I was more interested in their lives than in this Tolkien-like world I was attempting to create. I listened to their conversations, wishing I could join in with my views on designer clothes — not that I had much to add, mind you! Thus ended my alternate life as a mole-like hero in my dream world.

I regretted all the times I'd ignored Jill in the past, my nose stuck in the newspaper as she told me about her day. How I wished I was back there now. My heart leaped for joy whenever she came to see me in the NICU. I delighted in her telling me about the kids, what the doctor had said, which friend had sent supper over, what the day was like. On some days, her presence was all I had to look forward to.

It was strange to have my children see me defenceless and vulnerable. Not that I had ever tried to pretend I was invincible, but I was the dad. They told me about school, what they were reading or doing, things a dad wants to hear. My brother, Duane, was constantly at my side. My stepfather, Ron (whom I called Dad), and my mom were frequent visitors, and they were good companions for Jill in those first few weeks.

My mother gave me my first laugh. A priest, whose mother was a patient of mine, came to visit me. He was dressed in his priestly attire, as he had probably just visited a sick parishioner in hospital. My mother, who was quite anxious and distraught over my condition, saw the priest at my bedside and jumped to conclusions. She took him aside — out of my hearing, she thought — and said, "Father, you aren't giving him the last rites, are you?" If I had been capable of making a sound, they would have heard a loud guffaw.

It was strange also to have my friends, fellow doctors, suddenly become my caregivers. Yet I felt uplifted and reassured by their visits. Was this how my patients felt when I visited them?

The Saint John Regional Hospital is located on a hill outside of the city's central business section, in a forested area, and the NICU is on the fourth floor. I oriented myself in the NICU by imagining I was in a long corridor. Yet I knew this couldn't be true. I had visited patients in the NICU many times in the past. I knew it was square, with patients arranged along one wall opposite the nursing desk and another to the left. It was spacious and kept dimly lit. The windows, which didn't open to the outside air, were narrow and faced south. I was aware of other patients on either side of me, but I could not shake the notion that I was in a narrow room with patients aligned down one side.

Adding to my disorientation was the fact that I could not move my neck; I could look only in the direction the nurses placed me. When they cautiously raised my head (they were afraid it would cause dizziness), I could make out the nursing desk. The inability to look around frustrated me! I had double vision because the muscles in my eyeballs were not working together. The nerves that control these muscles arise from the brainstem nuclei. My glasses compounded my problems with orientation. They were progressive bifocals; the bottom half was for reading. While on my back, I could look out of only the bottom half, so everything was blurred. My view of the ceiling was great, though I believe I saw double the number of dots in the tiles.

I later met a fellow in my community who had sustained a brainstem stroke a year before me. His double vision, or diplopia, never improved. He wore an eye patch to stop it.

I started to suffer from headaches, which I supposed were brought on by these vision problems. They didn't last too long into my convalescence, but they were another problem I didn't need. I felt like a futuristic portrait of mankind, all brain and no body. But I did know I had a body. How it was misbehaving!

Depression crept in. Darkness, black loneliness, the frustration of being unable to just get up, of being forced to lie there against my will, my own body holding me captive. I wanted to go home with Jill, sit in my favourite chair and read my paper, watch a movie with my children, anything but lie there.

My worst day was the first Sunday, three days after my stroke, when the staff decided to get me up. Instead of relief, my first time out of bed was filled with sadness.

First, an extension from a specialized chair was slid under me, which then lifted me up and onto the seat. The nurses carefully brought the chair up from horizontal to a very slight upright position. I looked outside and saw a clear blue sky, with trees gently swaying in the wind. The parking lot was pretty much empty, reminding me that most people were home on this late Sunday afternoon. Normally I would have been at the cottage, getting ready to depart for our home in town. I would have felt refreshed and recharged, anticipating a new week. Instead, I lay there wishing I could feel that breeze, the fresh air. It made me feel so blue. I missed Jill and my children. A feeling of unreality pervaded my soul. *This can't be happening!*

I never cried during those first few weeks. I seemed to be emotionally comatose. It was as though this sudden change, from being a healthy caregiver to an invalid, was too much for my brain to comprehend.

A nurse mistakenly thought I was crying when my eyes were tearing from some irritation. "Are you thinking too much?" she asked as she tenderly wiped the tears from my face.

I'm not crying! My eyes are burning out of my head! I tried to scream.

"Don't think. Try to rest. Let each day go by. And who knows?"

I know. My eyes are about to explode!

Throughout this ordeal, my face was expressionless. No one could tell from my face that I was in pain. The nurse was caring and I accepted her sympathy. I welcomed it, but I welcomed more the cool, wet towel she eventually got for my eyes.

No one could read my face. My brother-in-law, Ted, bestowed on me a most beautiful discourse about my virtues and what I meant to him. All the while, I was dying with a headache.

A week went by. I was surviving on IV fluid, but this could not continue; I would need food. Because I was unable to swallow, a feeding tube had to be inserted. For long-term use, the best type is a gastrostomy tube that is inserted into the stomach through the abdominal wall. The end inside the stomach has an inflatable bulb that prevents it from slipping out. Liquid supplements are given through the open end and can be used to sustain a person indefinitely.

The time had also come for my endotracheal tube to be removed. This type of tube sticks out of the patient's mouth and goes down the windpipe, or trachea. If it remains in the trachea too long, ulcers will form, leading to infection and ultimately the breakdown of the air passages, a life-threatening situation. I was off the respirator, yet I couldn't be trusted to breathe on my own because my epiglottis, the valve on the top of the trachea that prevents fluid and food from entering the lungs, was not working. Without a tube, I would be aspirating saliva, food that I burped up from the tube feedings, and gastric juices. My lungs had to be protected. Besides, my breathing muscles were not strong enough to pull air into my lungs.

It requires much less energy to breathe through a hole in your throat. As the neurologist had told my family, I would need a tracheotomy to insert a tube into my trachea below my larynx, or voice box. A tracheotomy tube, or trach for short, has an inflatable bulb on one end that prevents debris from entering the lungs, completely sealing off the lungs from the outside.

I was taken to the operating room for the insertion of both the feeding tube and the trach about a week after I entered the NICU. Everything went well, except I had a big problem: without the endotracheal tube in my mouth, I bit down on my tongue. My chewing muscles were set to *on*. The signal from my spinal cord telling the muscles to relax was not getting through. My jaws were clenched tight and, unfortunately, my tongue ended up between my teeth.

The nurses tried putting in an oral airway. This is a plastic device that goes from the patient's mouth to the back of the throat. But my jaw was so tightly clenched that no manner of twisting, prodding, or force could get that oral airway between my teeth. Besides, trying was hurting my tongue. Then the nurses decided to try tongue depressors. They succeeded in wedging in some depressors after many attempts, but at a cost to my tongue. I dreaded the moment I saw them come with more tongue depressors.

"I think we'll give it another try, Shawn," a nurse said.

Leave me alone! My tongue is fine! I tried to cry.

I was wrong. Jill later told me they had to do something; my tongue was grossly swollen and had turned blue and yellow. Why didn't I feel this? I have no idea.

But the tongue depressors wouldn't stay in place. We needed a more permanent solution. Someone came up with the idea of dental clamps, which are used to keep a patient's mouth open during dental surgery. Who better to put them in but my dentist? He came in one evening, gave me a muscle relaxant through my IV, and put the clamp in place. It worked — and apparently I looked quite the sight!

That dental clamp remained sticking out of my mouth for days. Another dentist switched it to the other side of my mouth to prevent mouth ulcers. A few days after that, I yawned and the clamp fell out for good. I would spend months trying to open my mouth farther.

One day, a speech language pathologist came in with what he called an eye-gaze board. Before this, he had been trying to stimulate my swallowing with metal instruments that he immersed in ice and then applied to the back of my throat. I could swallow reflexively, but I could not initiate one voluntarily. Jill was encouraged each time I swallowed, but I could tell by the speech language pathologist's reaction that he was not very impressed.

Suspicious of this eye-gaze board, I listened to his explanation of how to use it. I thought, *I will be a good patient and humour him. I'll learn how to use it, but I won't need it long. I'll be talking soon, once they remove this trach, which will be soon. I'll be singing.*

It was easy enough to understand how to use the board. The eye-gaze board was clear plastic with a hole in the centre through which the person with whom I was conversing looked at me. Around the hole facing me were eight cards with letters of the alphabet, numbers, or short phrases. I looked at the card where the letter or number I wanted was located. The person watched my eyes to direct them to the duplicate card on their side of the board. When the correct card was chosen, we proceeded to find the correct letter or number. On each card the letters or numbers were arranged exactly like the cards on the board, so instead of looking at that card, I pretended the board was that card only and gazed in the direction on the board where it would appear on the card. It sounds complicated but it wasn't, though it was painfully slow.

Before long, the speech language pathologist and I were having our first conversation. Significantly, one of the first things I asked him was "When will I be able to talk?"

His answer was evasive. I expected him to say, "Maybe a couple of weeks, Shawn." Instead he said, "A while."

What does that mean? Of course he can't say anything; he isn't my doctor. Why is everybody being so careful?

I was familiar with the health care world. No one likes to take responsibility, because they may say the wrong thing. This was what I thought was happening. To some extent that was true, but really, they knew I needed time to slowly adjust to my new life. I was in the first stage of loss: denial. Everyone needs to go through the five stages of loss: denial, anger, bargaining, depression, and acceptance. People can be gently supported through these stages, but there is no shortcut. Denial is a necessary psychological defensive mechanism; the brain needs it when the truth is too hard to accept.

Jill took to the eye-gaze board eagerly. It was great to finally be able to converse with her. It wasn't easy, though. Because my eyes did not move together, it was hard for the person I was talking with to follow them. Which eye were they to follow? Letter by letter, Jill and I would plod along. The conversations had to be kept short and superficial. Before long, my eyes would get teary from the strain of trying to control their muscles.

My parents found it difficult to use the eye-gaze board. My mother would later tell me that her heart was never really in it because she, like me, thought I would be talking before long. And the eye-gaze board wasn't useful for interacting with the nurses because most of them weren't familiar with it.

Now that I was off the respirator, I was ready to leave the NICU. My first big step in recovery! I had been in the unit for twelve days. Those nights, those days — they all ran together. When I learned I would be leaving, I felt like screaming, *"Now we're getting somewhere!"*

CHAPTER 6
THE FLOOR

I was introduced to my new room, a ward of four beds. The wall between the room and the corridor was all glass and the room was located beside the nursing desk so we could be observed.

I had achieved my first step toward complete recovery by being released from the NICU. I had no idea, as I settled into my new room, how difficult that journey would be and how unrealistic my expectations were.

I was delighted to be placed next to one of the windows and to have a television. I had spent the last twelve days looking at the ceiling, listening to fragments of conversations, watching the nurses as they came into my field of vision, and enduring my endless thoughts. Television would be a welcome diversion.

A major disappointment. I could not get comfortable to watch TV. When someone did manage to get me into a comfortable position, my double vision thwarted my pursuit of a pleasurable experience. Even when I corrected my diplopia by covering one eye, I was disinterested in what was on TV. I looked upon news and sports, things I used to enjoy, with indifference. Were my physical disabilities frustrating me and preventing me from enjoying TV, or was it my mental state?

Lack of concentration, insomnia, and the inability to enjoy simple pleasures are symptoms of depression. I had reason to be depressed, but I didn't *feel* depressed.

On the floor, I became more aware of and interested in my surroundings and life around me. The man beside me was confused and kept trying to get out of bed. His family was attentive and stayed by his side. I thought I smiled when they looked over at me, inviting a comment, but my face was not expressing my intent. Little wonder I received no response. I must have looked like I was brain dead, alive but not really aware. At that point, it didn't occur to me how people might perceive me. I felt the same inside as I always had.

Pain was still ever present. Now that I was out of the NICU, the nurses could spend less time with me, and I had a whole new group to educate about the meaning of my furious blinking. Most of them knew to look at me, but occasionally some didn't; they did their job and left. That was very frustrating and disappointing.

Moving my leg was usually all that was necessary to resolve the pain. However, within minutes the pain would be back in a different spot in the same leg. So perhaps it didn't really matter whether anyone helped me move, because the pain would soon be returning. But any relief was so appreciated, even if it was only for a few minutes. I'm not sure why I didn't request more mild pain-killers — not even acetaminophen. I was still playing the tough, macho doctor role, I guess.

Sleep was difficult. I longed for a break from the constant thinking, the pain in my legs, and my blurred vision. I wanted to wake up refreshed after a good eight hours of sleep.

The reticular activating system, responsible for the act of falling asleep, is located in the brainstem and can be affected by an injury to this area. In my case, it definitely was altered. I spent countless hours just staring at the drapes. I would catnap throughout the night. The doctors tried me on mild sedatives, but they had no effect. I went for weeks with little sleep. It was not worth the effort, at 3:00 a.m., to tell a nurse I wasn't sleeping. What could they do? Better to try again with another medication the next night.

Instead, I watched the sitter read while I played mind games and battled with my thoughts. The hospital hired people just to sit and watch over me during the night because I wasn't able to ring a bell for help and they were still uncomfortable about my breathing. But it wasn't very practical; in the dark, it was impossible for the sitters to see me blink my eyelids for help. Most of the time, I just gave up.

It was strange to be so close to the sitters, night after night, and never talk. I would experience this feeling many times in the months to come. I enjoyed talking to people; it was what I did every day. I had grown from a shy young man to a confident person who welcomed conversation. I wanted to ask the sitters about university, their families, sports, anything.

I was alone with my thoughts.

I thought of Jill, my children, my parents, and my patients. I had learned so much over the twenty years of my medical practice — so many lives and stories, so much pain and love. I had many memories to keep me entertained.

CHAPTER 7
KATHLEEN

I took over an existing family practice from a well-liked doctor. He had started his practice after serving in the Second World War, and over the years, he had developed quite a following of patients who were all very fond of him. When he retired, he asked me to take over his practice. I was fresh out of medical school and my internship. His patients, who were sorry to see their beloved doctor go, probably anticipated that I would change things, screw up their medications, never be available, and God knows what else.

I did initiate many changes, but I also adjusted to their expectations. His patients and I, for the most part, gradually grew to accept each other, and thus began twenty years of wonderful relationships. In medical school, we had been warned that a doctor can't afford to get too involved in the lives or feelings of patients. The transference of feelings can weigh too heavily on caregivers, so to remain strong, they have to learn to divorce themselves from what their patients are experiencing emotionally and physically. Caregivers will do their patients no good if they get sick, too, and many caregivers struggle with their own wellness because of emotional transference.

I struggled with this at first but eventually found a balance between empathy and emotional transference. But I had a hard time preventing a strong emotional bond forming with some patients.

Kathleen was in her nineties. She was thin, grey haired, and frail, but mentally very sharp. She lived with her daughter, who was in her seventies, in an affordable apartment complex. I made home visits to her because her health was too poor to allow her to come to my office, and I began to look forward to our encounters. She enthralled me with tales of her life, her husband, and the city in earlier years. She didn't complain much, but I could see her breathing was becoming more laboured over time. She was dying of heart failure, and all the drugs in the world were not going to help her tired, old heart.

She made me laugh. I was comfortable in her presence and I fell in love with her. She had me wrapped around her little finger.

One day, while I was working in my office, I got a call from Kathleen. She said she was short of breath and asked if I could come to see her. I told her that of course I would, but it would be a few hours. I had an office full of patients and I was booked for the whole day. All seemed well at that point.

The day was going by quickly when I received another call from Kathleen. I could tell from her voice that things were not right. She had called back to tell me her breathing was worse. I could hear the unmistakable sound of someone in pulmonary edema, a condition in which fluid backs up in the lungs because of a failing heart. I told her I was calling an ambulance, right then, to take her to hospital. She begged me not to call and told me she was all right; she would wait until I could come.

I reluctantly agreed to her request, but I felt uneasy. As I finished with the patients remaining in my waiting room, I kept thinking that I should have been more forceful with her. I shouldn't have let Kathleen talk me into letting her stay home.

I finally left my office in haste after my last patient. As I approached her apartment building, I saw her daughter watching out for me from the front window.

I heard Kathleen before I saw her. Her breathing was laboured and her colour ashen. I knew before I placed my stethoscope on her back that I would hear bubbling sounds throughout her lungs. She was in massive pulmonary edema. Her heart was beating in a regular, slow rhythm, but the pumping action of the heart was failing. If she were to get through this, she would need IV furosemide, a diuretic drug used to flush fluid out of the body.

"Do I have to go? I hate the hospital," she said between breaths.

I chastised her. "I need to give you a drug through an IV to make you pee out fluid. You should have gone to hospital when I said."

"If you say so, Doc."

"I know so. It's the only way to get you comfortable."

I waited with her until the ambulance arrived and then followed them to the hospital, where I examined her again in the ER and wrote the orders and admission history. All seemed well. The diuretic had started to work by the time I left. I joked with her about something silly and left rather satisfied that Kathleen would soon be feeling better.

I was late getting home that evening. We were still living in an apartment on the east side of Saint John. I had been home only about half an hour when the ER doctor called.

"I know you're not on call," he said, "but I thought you would want to know. The patient you admitted tonight has just passed away."

"*What?*"

"She was doing fine and the nurses were just about to take her up to the floor, when she stopped breathing. Appears that her heart just stopped. You had a no-code order, so I just pronounced her."

A no-code order is an order not to use CPR to resuscitate a patient whose heart has stopped. The ER doctor had pronounced her dead.

"Is her daughter still there?" I asked.

"Yeah, she was right beside her when she took her last breath. Talking right up until the end, apparently."

"Can I talk to her?"

I said the usual: "I'm sorry," "tried my best," "guess her heart was too old," "going to miss her." After I hung up, I started to cry. Bewildered, I went into my bedroom, lay down, and sobbed.

I cried over losing her. I cried because I had thought I would save her. I was frustrated and tired. Jill consoled me, although she probably thought it was a strange reaction; she had never seen me react to a patient's death like this before. But I had broken the rule with Kathleen and had become too close.

I would never again cry over losing a patient. I learned my lesson: There needs to be a wall between the doctor and the patient. I always felt close to my patients, but after that I never forgot that they were patients, not friends. This wall protected me and prevented emotional strain. But it also benefitted my patients. Doctors don't make good clinical judgments when they are too emotionally invested in their patients. A caregiver can still be very empathetic while not sharing the patient's emotional reaction to life-changing events.

Still, this would remain a struggle. It was hard not to become immersed in a patient's joy or sorrow after knowing them for twenty years.

CHAPTER 8
PREPARING

My tube feedings had started when I was in the NICU. A specific amount of liquid supplement was syringed directly into my stomach tube, a method called bolus feeding. The amount seemed to have no effect on how I felt; it made me neither full nor hungry. However, as a result of the feedings, by the time I was on the floor, the nurses decided I needed to have a bowel movement. I don't know what type of suppository they used, but it caused excruciating cramps. It could have been that I didn't need to go or I was constipated or I was sensitive to that type of suppository. I don't know what the problem was, but it was my first taste of being a *real* patient.

As the suppository worked, they placed a sheet under my bum and told me I was to defecate on it. A novel experience! I never imagined I could do such a thing, but I had no choice. I swallowed my pride and let nature take its course. I hated having a bowel movement in bed, but it would be months before I could sit up. Eventually, they found a type of suppository that didn't cause so much cramping.

Another duty the nurses carried out with military precision was turning me. I was turned every two hours to prevent bedsores and to increase comfort. This probably didn't help my sleep, but I welcomed it; it relieved my aches and pains, if only temporarily.

The catheter had been removed from my bladder in the NICU just before I left and I was using a condom catheter that was attached to a drainage bag.

When I was in the NICU, the occupational therapist fashioned splints for my arms and legs. When there has been an injury to the brainstem, the arms and hands tend to go into a flexed, contracted position and the legs and feet tend to become extended. Splints are used to try to prevent this from becoming permanent. Having both arms and legs splinted for two hours on and two hours off day and night was uncomfortable and hot. I knew the splints were necessary, but that didn't make wearing them any easier.

Physiotherapists started stretching exercises while I was in the NICU. My knees would be flexed high onto my chest and my arms stretched high over my head. *There*, I thought. *Certainly they can see I am supple and my recovery will be quick. I bet they're amazed at how good I am!*

I was denying the truth: in any spinal injury there is a period of spinal shock during which the muscles are flaccid before they become rigid. My being supple during this period was expected, but I wanted to believe I was going to recover more quickly than they anticipated. I thought I would astound them. Instead, I astounded myself.

One day, the neurologist asked me if I would be willing to go to Stan Cassidy Centre for Rehabilitation, the tertiary-care centre for rehabilitation in the province. It is located in Fredericton, the capital city of New Brunswick, a little more than an hour's drive from Saint John. I agreed. The transfer would happen soon.

Before this transfer occurred, I had a magnetic resonance image (MRI) scan. The head nurse of the neurological floor, whom I knew quite well professionally and socially, came with me. It felt strange to lie on a stretcher being wheeled through the familiar corridors, watching the lights and ceiling tiles pass by over my head, seeing staff I had interacted with a scant week before. Now I was the patient.

The MRI machine was small and noisy; the banging seemed out of place for such a precise techno-machine. During an MRI, the patient spends a fair amount of time inside the machine. I imagined rhythms based on the fans circulating air in the unit. The nurse stayed outside, watching my trach tube for congestion in case it needed suctioning.

The MRI showed the infarction, or area of cell death, to be on the pons, a part of the brainstem that looks like a walnut. It measured twenty-one millimetres by twelve millimetres — less than an inch long and about half an inch deep. It's hard to conceive that such a small area can cause such devastation. As well, a small linear area had died on my cerebellum, an appendage on the base of the brain that looks like a slice of cauliflower and is used mainly for balance.

The area of cell death on my pons was close to the respiratory centre, so I knew I was lucky to be alive. But my life would change dramatically owing to that twenty-one millimetres, a pathetically small injury for destroying a multitude of dreams. It didn't seem right.

That same day, another nurse friend who worked on the neurological floor took my mother and Jill to see the Stan Cassidy Centre for Rehabilitation. They felt comfortable with the staff, but they were surprised at how small and old the building was.

Meanwhile, I was having problems with my ears again. I have had hearing problems since I was a little boy. It seemed to start from a deviated septum or from breaking my nose while playing hockey. I also had allergies that caused excessive mucus production, which in turn blocked my auditory tubes. As a result of all this, I experienced repeated ear infections, which led to scarring of my eardrums.

I felt another earache developing. Besides the pain, I became deaf as more fluid built up in my middle ear. I could not hear anyone speak. For a few days, I experienced what it must be like to be speech impaired and deaf. I worried that being unable to hear my therapist's instructions would slow my recovery.

The same otolaryngologist who had lanced my eardrum before my stroke came to my rescue the day before I left the Regional. For some reason, he had to replace my trach tube, and while he was doing this, he replaced my eardrum tubes, which were blocked after being in place for only two weeks. Now I could hear things I hadn't heard in years. I probably should have gotten eardrum tubes years before, but I was always "too busy."

I felt no anxiety as I was wheeled to the operating room for this surgery. After all, how could things get worse? I simply fell asleep once the anesthetist gave me his magic needle, and then I woke up in recovery. Again, I marvelled at my lack of concern. Normally, I would have experienced some anxiety symptoms, like abdominal cramps, sweaty palms, and maybe some light-headedness before surgery. But I was calm, unconcerned, and cool.

The next day, I was ready to leave the Regional for Stan Cassidy. It had been more than two weeks since my stroke, and I was eager to go. Friends and nurses came to say goodbye. I lifted my left thumb up in response to their encouragement. My left thumb was the first of my limbs to regain movement. I expected my right thumb would start moving shortly. Eighteen months later, I still couldn't move my right thumb.

It was a beautiful Monday morning when I left Saint John for Fredericton. I was to be transported by ambulance, and for the first time, I felt a twinge of anxiety. My trach got congested periodically and required suctioning, a hideous but necessary procedure. Did the ambulance attendant know how to do that? Would I get into respiratory trouble during my trip? (Of course the attendant could do that; he was a young paramedic who probably knew how to manage an airway much better than I did.) With these questions, I left the hospital. I was sure I wouldn't be at the rehab centre long. I'm glad I didn't know the truth.

CHAPTER 9
THE TRANSFER

It was the hottest May 31 we'd ever had. Great! I spent it in the back of an ambulance, with no air conditioning, wrapped up in blankets and breathing through a tube in my neck!

I was impressed at how clean the back of the ambulance was. I was able to see the sky out of the back window, so I amused myself by trying to determine our position on the highway by the turns and hills the ambulance took. *Now we're going along Harbour Bridge. Should be stopping soon at the toll booth.* I verified whether I was right by watching out for landmarks high enough for me to see out the window as we passed by.

The closer we got to Fredericton, the hotter it became. I heard the ambulance attendants comment and grumble about the air conditioning not working.

Sweat rolled into my eye. The paramedic tried to make me comfortable, but how could I tell him my eyes were burning? It is amazing to me now how I endured these minor irritations. How often does your scalp or nose itch, your mouth get a little too moist, a fleck of skin land on your eyelash — little things you can take care of with a quick touch or rub with your fingers? A lot! I had to accept and endure them and be content with the knowledge that eventually that itch or other sensory annoyance would go away.

It was not really that simple. Sometimes enduring the irritation was torturous and I tried to get my mind off it by refocusing my thoughts on other things. On this trip, with my eyes burning, my mind drifted again to my past experiences.

The ER was always an adventure. For many years, general practitioners in our area were required to work ER shifts, and I did this for twelve years, until the requirement was lifted. By then, a new breed of doctor had emerged, the emergentologist, and as more of them moved into our community, I felt it was a good time to leave the ER and concentrate on my family practice.

Emergency medicine can make a health care professional feel great one minute and terrible the next. There is no time to recuperate between a tragedy and the next patient. The same holds true in the office, but at a slower pace. I often had to inform a patient they had cancer and deal with that emotional trauma and then, within a few minutes and with no chance to reflect, give my full attention to a child.

The adrenalin rush in the ER — from cardiac arrests, multiple traumas, and other urgent cases — can be addictive. There is no greater high than success, and no greater low than failure. I feared that I might order the wrong thing, forget something, freeze, or be the factor that cost a life. Thankfully, that never happened.

Not all ER work is urgent; about 75 percent of cases are minor problems: colds, earaches, cuts, sprains, and an odd assortment of other ailments. Even when I wasn't confronted with life-threatening emergencies, the hustle and bustle of emergency work caused its own adrenalin rush. In fact, I could not go home and simply fall asleep. I had to unwind first, no matter how tired I was.

One night that sticks in my memory was when a bus over-turned on the highway. I was terrified by the confusion and may-hem of suddenly being confronted with thirteen victims. I called in a lot of help that night.

The worst night, however, was when a young drunk driver collided with two women and their children who were on the way to a Halloween party. He drove up an off-ramp the wrong way and smashed into the car containing the two moms and their chil-dren as they were driving down the highway exit. I could imagine the horror they felt as they saw what was about to happen but had no way to avoid the collision. The young man was the first one brought into the ER. He was drunk and pretty badly broken up, with multiple fractures, lacerations, and possible internal damage. He was conscious and yelling like a banshee.

We learned that the young mother who was driving died at the scene, but the passengers were stable and had suffered only minor injuries. The young girl whose mother had died was car-ried into the trauma room by her dad, a policeman. Can you imagine being called to the scene of an accident and finding your wife and daughter? The sight of this policeman carrying in his little girl, knowing his wife had just died, was so tragic.

The drunk driver chose that moment to cry out for his mother. "Mommy, Mommy!" he yelled in a loud, sobbing voice.

I wouldn't have been surprised if the policeman had drawn his revolver and shot the guy. To his credit, he said nothing. He quietly spoke to his daughter while the nurses took them to another area. For the first and only time in my career, I felt like harming a patient. I fought the urge to "mistakenly" lean on his broken leg or get caught up in his urinary catheter or IV and pull it out. The more he wailed, the more I wanted to hurt him.

I didn't. Eventually we stabilized him and sent him to the operating room. I never forgot that cold night, the policeman and his daughter, or my anger. Similar scenarios still happen too often. Drunk driving has to be dealt with harshly; it is intolerable.

The heat in the back of the ambulance was intolerable. My eyes were still burning from the sweat seeping from my forehead. *If only I could get this blanket off me.* I searched for the paramedic's eyes, and when he finally looked at me, I frantically blinked. He looked away. *Of course, he doesn't understand the way I communicate. This is hopeless. Wouldn't it be common sense to anyone to remove this blanket in this heat?*

I resigned myself to the torture and tried to focus on something else. Eventually, my eyes somehow stopped burning and we arrived at Stan Cassidy Centre for Rehabilitation.

Jill told me later that she thought something bad must have happened during the trip, because as they pulled my stretcher out the back door of the ambulance, my face looked so sweaty and pale and my hair was so wet.

The air felt good. It was the first time I had felt fresh air since my stroke. Unfortunately, the pleasure was short lived, because the paramedics quickly wheeled me through the front doors.

CHAPTER 10
STAN CASSIDY CENTRE
FOR REHABILITATION

I was shocked by the appearance of the centre. I had expected the tertiary-care centre for rehabilitative medicine for the province of New Brunswick to be a modern facility; instead it was a low, white-cement building, and obviously old.

My immediate impression that it looked like something from the 1950s was confirmed when I spotted a stone just outside the front door inscribed with a 1957 date. Two people from Saint John greeted me at the front door as I was wheeled through. One was an old friend, and it struck me how improbable it was that she and I should end up here at the same time, in a rehabilitation centre far from home.

She had suffered spinal cord trauma from a motor vehicle accident. At that point, no one knew how much function she would regain. She had been extremely lucky to escape with her life. Even luckier still, most of her leg function would return in time. We had grown up in a small summertime community called Sand Point, and I had just visited her on the neurological floor of the Saint John Regional Hospital about a week before my stroke.

The man from Saint John was completely paralyzed from the neck down as a rare complication of a viral infection. It would take more than a year, but eventually he would regain good use of his hands and be able to walk with a cane.

They greeted me outside the entrance to the cafeteria. The walls inside the building were made of the same white cement blocks as those outside, giving the whole area a cold feel. As I passed the cafeteria, I saw they had tried to warm it up with different colours and cheerful decorations, but that didn't hide the fact the walls were cement blocks.

I was whisked down a corridor, had a quick stop at the nurses' desk, and then on to my room, number 8. The walls were the same white-cement blocks. The outer wall had many windows looking out onto a courtyard, which was enclosed on three sides by the building and featured a gazebo in the centre. Perennials and shrubs — sadly, not maintained or weeded — lined the walls outside. This state of neglect, I would come to understand, symbolized the financial strain that rehabilitative medicine was under in this province.

My room had a sink, and in a little room off to the side there was a toilet — which I would never use. A closet was located on the same wall as the toilet room and the sink.

I was shocked at these conditions. I had worked all my life in a modern hospital setting. I tried not to show it; I tried to make the best of it, but I was disappointed.

That down feeling did not last long, because in came the head nurse. Louise was a young British woman with long, blond hair, and she projected a sunny, confident personality from the start. I was astounded that this young woman could be the head nurse. Over the coming months, I grew to appreciate her and understand why she had this role. She was amazingly strong for her build and could single-handedly swing me from my bed to a chair. She owned a farm and enthralled me with stories of her goat, who had a nasty habit of butting gentlemen callers. Perhaps that was why she was still single.

After introductions and the arranging of my room, she began to wash me because of my sweaty journey. My face, then my chest, then over onto one side to do my back. Then she said, in her British accent, "Now it's time to do your nooks and crannies!"

My mind quickly scrolled through all the anatomy I knew. *Must be an English thing. Behind the ears? No. The armpits? No. The toes? That's it! No. Oh no! It can't be!*

To my horror and before I could think much more, my diaper was off and there I was, exposed and vulnerable. Without a word from either of us, soap and water were slapped on and I was dried and diapered before I had time to be embarrassed.

It soon became routine. There is no place for modesty in the disabled world. I had to get used to the idea of having strangers invade my private person. The bed baths, my genitalia washed twice a day, the bowel routine, having my bum wiped, putting on a condom catheter — all necessary, but so hard to endure at first. For me, having someone else wipe my bum was the hardest personal act to get used to. But I knew the nurses were professionals and this was part of their job, so I never felt I lost my dignity.

After my introduction to Stan Cassidy and the head nurse, other nurses took off my regulation hospital wear and dressed me in street clothes. I was surprised, but already I felt positive about this; it was my first step toward rehabilitation.

Within a few hours, an occupational therapist brought in a wheelchair. She transferred me into the chair with a lift. I lay, rather than sat, in my chair, which had a headrest for my wobbly head. At this point I could not hold up my head, but it would become one of the first things I could do. They were afraid I might become dizzy and nauseated getting up and moving, but I didn't. It felt good to finally be mobile. Mom and Jill took me outside that afternoon.

I couldn't turn my head or see much, but the air felt good. I closed my eyes and breathed in, finally free of those institutional smells. I savoured the warmth of the sun on my skin and the sounds of wind moving through trees, cars going by, and people talking — normal sounds and smells and sensations. The people around me talked about common things, things that weren't about me, a world other than sickness. It felt so good!

My time outside quickly ended, and soon I was back in bed. At the Regional, I had been accustomed to continuous humidity for my trach. Here, I was introduced to intermittent humidity. Humidity is moisture given through the breathed-in air to keep the lungs moist. At Stan Cassidy, they used some archaic device from years back, which surprised me. A nebulizer, like a small plastic cup, was hooked into a hollow tube that ran from my trach to a small air compressor that was noisy and looked old. The nebulizer was tricky; it had to be held a certain way or it wouldn't work, and because I had no hand control, the nebulizer treatment often took longer than necessary to finish.

If you wanted humidified air at the Regional, or any modern care facility, you just plugged your mask tube into the wall and adjusted the flow. I had trained and worked at modern hospitals all my life; Stan Cassidy was looking poor to me so far. They were supposed to help me?

If I thought the aerosol machines were old, I had a greater shock when I saw the condition of the suction machines. At the Regional, suction outlets were on the wall in every room and the degree of suctioning could be adjusted as needed. At Stan Cassidy, they brought in a type of suction device I hadn't seen in years. This baby was ancient and noisy.

Rather than use the bolus feeding method I'd had at the Regional, the nutritionist at Stan Cassidy decided to use what is called continuous feeds. This is done with a machine that regulates the rate at which the liquid flows in through the gastrostomy tube. Finally, a device I was quite familiar with, and state of the art.

I had expected so much more from Stan Cassidy than I was seeing. I ended my first day with a heavy heart. But this blue feeling was counteracted by news that Jill would be staying with me for the first night in a bed set up beside me. It was exciting, like having a sleepover when we were kids. It would have been so nice to talk with Jill, eat popcorn, watch a movie, maybe hold hands, but none of that could happen. I was content enough to have her in the same room.

The health staff didn't trust my breathing; they were afraid I might suddenly stop breathing owing to the damage to my brainstem. The neurologist in Saint John had arranged for an apneic device to be attached to my chest. I bet it was more to reassure Jill than to a real probability that I would need it. The device would ring an alarm if I stopped breathing. After a few nights of alarms ringing for no reason, I asked them to give it up. By this time, sleep was more important to me than breathing.

My first day at rehab ended with mixed feelings. I was happy to have Jill at my side, happy to be on the road to recovery, but disappointed in the Stan Cassidy Centre. I was soon to learn that there was more to Stan Cassidy than met the eye. The next day I was introduced to my physiotherapist, occupational therapist, and speech language pathologist. They became my whole life. For the next ten months, they were my daily routine. They were my world. They were my hope.

CHAPTER 11
REALITY AND ANGER

In the early part of June, I was still in denial. By this time I had conceded that it might take the whole summer to rehabilitate before I'd be ready to return to work in the fall. It never entered my mind that I might not be able to return to my family practice as before.

Jill or my mother often stayed at Kiwanis House, low-cost accommodations provided by Stan Cassidy for families of patients, located just behind the centre. They vowed I would not be left alone because of my helplessness.

Jill or Mom would often wheel me out to the courtyard and read to me in the gazebo. I was hot because of the diaper and the white antiembolic stockings, which prevented blood clots, and again my eyes frequently burned. The diplopia blurring my surroundings, the drastic lifestyle changes, and my helplessness made these moments feel surreal. However, despite all of that, it was wonderful to be outside. Spending a pleasant hour there with Jill or Mom reading to me, I could lose myself for a short time, a welcome relief from the reality of being locked in.

There was a park beside the centre featuring huge weeping willows, a gravel pathway, areas for barbecues, another gazebo, and two small bridges over a marsh. I loved to sit under a huge willow tree, feeling the branches touch my face, and gaze upon the marsh, hoping to see a frog resting in the shallows. Dragonflies flew randomly through the reeds. I felt as though I could be happy here. Perhaps, I thought, I would soon be able to spend contented hours here gardening, taking pictures, or just reading.

But my hopeful contemplations were always destroyed by some physical symptom: my bum aching for relief from the wheelchair seat, my trach becoming congested, or a headache developing from the double vision. What was I thinking? I couldn't stay away for any length of time before I needed nursing assistance. I guess I saw potential in this park as a place to get away from the daily nursing routine, a little area to fulfill my need for independence and solitude, a place I could practise my improving muscle function. It never happened.

Like the centre itself, the park was the victim of underfinancing. The gazebo and firepit needed repairs, and only weeds grew in the flower pots. Patients seldom used the park; most of us were too beaten up in body or spirit to enjoy it. But it was a welcome reprieve for me even if my visits were short.

My independence was seriously curtailed by the need to have my trach tube cleared of phlegm, which was being overly produced owing to the tube irritating my trachea. I couldn't cough with enough force to discharge the phlegm myself. For some people, the trachea becomes used to the tube over time and the production of phlegm slows down, but in my case this never happened.

The procedure of suctioning started with a sterile, thin plastic tube being inserted down the trach tube into my windpipe. The plastic tube was hooked up to a suction machine that removed the phlegm, but in doing so it took all the air from my lungs. For a moment, I would feel as though I were suffocating. I involuntarily tried to breathe in against the machine, but at the same time, the suctioning tube caused a reflex cough because it was a foreign object in my trachea. There would be a moment of panic as my body tried to deal with opposing reflexes simultaneously, the urge to breathe in and to cough. This all occurred over a matter of seconds, but that knowledge didn't help me in that moment!

I was amazed to discover what the human body learned to tolerate. After a few months of this, I really didn't mind the suctioning. In fact, the phlegm rattling around in my trach tube was more bothersome than the procedure, and I often asked Jill or a nurse to suction my tube.

The day after my arrival at Stan Cassidy, I met the three therapists who became so very important to me. Beth was my speech language pathologist. I saw her twice a day, five days a week, as she helped me swallow again, then eat, make my first sounds, and finally, start to articulate. The tasks I had to do were always tedious and difficult and usually I failed, but I never gave up, mainly because of her humour, persistence, and faith in me.

Doreen was my occupational therapist. She was tall — although everyone looked tall from my wheelchair — and she wore a constant smile. Smiles were so important to me. She was instantly likeable and down to earth, with a huge laugh. She concentrated on my hands, transitioning from a sitting position to standing (called sit-to-stand), ability to move in bed, using a wheelchair, and adapting my environment to suit my disability. She was very intuitive; she knew when to push and when to back off. She expended a lot of energy on my behalf by setting up situations to challenge my body.

Mereille (pronounced *Mer-ay* to my Anglophone ear) was my physiotherapist. She was of average size and build, a francophone with a personality, attitude, and smile that were a constant source of reassurance to me. I gained strength from her enthusiasm over every small achievement. I also grew dependent on her; I watched her face for any small sign that I had achieved something or had done well. It became curiously important to me not to let her down. Mereille was very expressive, and her undying optimism about my recovery gave me the drive to improve and the attitude to never give up. Her greatest gift to me was hope.

These three women became my world for the next ten months, along with the nursing staff and my physiatrist, a doctor who specializes in rehabilitative medicine. Anything they said, I tried to do. I left my doctor's shingle at the front door. I didn't feel much like a physician anyway, so it wasn't hard.

My weekdays were pretty full with my three therapists. The nurses woke me at 6:00 a.m. to start my tube feeding so it would be over before my therapies started. I was washed and ready by 8:30. I usually started with speech therapy for half an hour, then physio-therapy for an hour, physiotherapy and occupational therapy combined for half an hour, and then finally occupational therapy alone for half an hour. Then it was time for lunch, which in my case was another can or two of that delicious tube feed. After lunch, I had another hour of physiotherapy, followed by another half hour of speech, and finally half an hour of occupational therapy. By this time it was 3:00 or 4:00 p.m. and I rested before "supper."

It sounds exhausting to me as I write about it now, but I was never that physically tired. Fatigue is very common after a stroke, and I was lucky that it was not too bad in my case. I prayed every night for strength.

My days were busy, with little time for introspection, but the weekends were another matter. The entire therapy staff was gone on weekends, so no treatments took place. Patients were encouraged to go home as part of their rehabilitation; only a few of us poor schmucks remained. The joint was dead! I had Jill, family, and friends with me, for which I'm forever grateful, but there were times when I had nothing but time.

I found it hard to keep my thoughts in the moment. I was dependent on others for every movement and function, and I couldn't easily interact with anyone for any length of time. So I ended up talking to myself, long conversations about everything and yet nothing. The act of talking to myself drove me crazy, but perhaps it gave me something to do and saved me from despair and depression.

As I said, I was still in denial and had not progressed from that first stage of loss, but on one of those boring weekends when I had too much time on my hands, that changed.

One afternoon, lying in my bed, I looked out the window at some tall pine trees bordering the property of Stan Cassidy. I was staring at these pines, enjoying their majestic appearance against the sky, when a crow happened to alight on a branch high up. I watched him skip from branch to branch. So effortless! His brain was so small, yet he performed manoeuvres I could only dream of. I couldn't even lift my hand. I was mad that I should be envious of a crow, yet enthralled with how marvellous nature and the simple things we take for granted truly were.

Reality hit me one day shortly after this incident, for no reason I could discern other than it was time: *I am locked in!* I said to myself. *I had a brainstem stroke. I may not improve. I could be like this for the rest of my life.*

This was reality: *I'm not at a summer retreat to get back in shape. I won't return to work in September. I probably won't return to work ever!*

Reality hit hard.

I fought the rising panic by thinking of Don, a patient of mine who was dying back home from cancer, and of Pauli, Ken, Joe, and other sick patients I had left in Saint John. Their reality was bleak, too. I was not alone.

I thought of what I would do with my practice. Would I sell it? It seemed so final, like I was abandoning all hope. I needed time.

I clung to hope. Hope that I would walk out of there. *I'm young,* I thought. *I can beat this thing.*

Once reality struck, anger was not far behind, but it did not last. I had the benefit of being an experienced doctor. For twenty years I had seen good people get struck down by disease and die for no good reason. I hated cancer. Despite trying my best to practise preventive medicine and be thorough in my screening procedures, cancer still beat my patients and me.

My patients rescued me from anger and the self-pity from which that emotion stems. I thought of Pauli with scleroderma, Don with lung cancer, Pat with Alzheimer's, and many more who were dying as I lay there. I saw before my eyes so many who had passed away over the last twenty years. Dave, such a gentle soul, who in his last days behaved so completely out of character due to the cancer that had spread to his brain. He would have been mortified by his own behaviour. It made it so hard for his family. So many deaths, so many ways to die. The memories of my patients and their courage saved me from prolonged anger and gave me strength.

Instead of asking "Why me?" I gradually realized this: "Why not me?" To think "Why me?" suggests I'm somehow special, that I deserve to be spared calamity.

I was never angry with God. I had long ago concluded that if God exists, he has no direct involvement in the day-to-day affairs of humans. That was the only way I could make sense of children dying, cancer, motor vehicle accidents, addictions, and other misfortunes. There may be a higher purpose to all the tragedies of mankind, as some religious people claim, but I can't embrace that philosophy and be expected to love God.

Thus, I went through denial, then quickly through anger and the why-me stages, lingered briefly in the what-ifs, and quietly arrived at acceptance. With acceptance, I became depressed. The depression was appropriate; how could anyone not become depressed in this situation? There are things I will never be able to do again, activities I loved. I mourned my losses.

I never became clinically depressed — although that is very common after a stroke. Rather, I felt blue. My depression manifested itself one sparkling June morning.

It was a Saturday, a bright, glorious day, and the nursing staff had prepared me for the day and transferred me into my wheelchair. I felt miserable, as I often did on beautiful days. Jill decided to wheel me outside for some fresh air. I saw a reflection of myself in the glass door on the way out. It was hard to imagine that was me. I didn't feel like that poor creature reflected in the mirror. Staring back at me was someone with the same blond hair but no expression on his face. *I am smiling, am I not?* His head was back, held up by a headrest. This fellow had a tube coming out of his throat with a white bandage around it. He wore my T-shirt and shorts, but he had on ridiculous-looking tight white stockings that stretched up past the bottom of his shorts. His abdomen stuck out. *I'm rather thin. I'm a runner.* My appearance only added to my sadness.

The air felt good as we wheeled out the sliding doors. Jill took me around the front and down the side of the building to the deck of Kiwanis House. It was already hot for 10:00 a.m. The birds were singing, the leaves rustling, the insects humming, and the more glorious and wonderful the day became, the more I drifted into despair.

I wanted so badly at that moment to stand up, to run among the trees, to lie down on the grass, to jump and laugh with wild abandonment for no other reason than I could. I couldn't spend the rest of my life like this, trapped inside a frozen body.

When we had settled on the deck, I made a motion with my eyes that I wanted to tell her something. Through the eye-gaze board I said, "Please kill me."

Jill was shocked, and with tears in her eyes she said, "Don't even think it!"

"Not now," I spelled. "No improvement, twelve months."

Although I felt like ending my life right then, I would give it more time. I had thought about it, and I didn't wish to live my life like this: unable to move my arms or legs, to smile, to speak, to eat — to partake of life. I had thought of how I would commit suicide. It would be impossible if I couldn't move; I would need help. Jill couldn't actively help me. Perhaps I could refuse the tube feedings.

A year later, I read about Jim, a man in his forties who had suffered a brainstem stroke. His wife interacted with brainstem stroke survivors on the internet. She told us about their struggles from the time he had the stroke. Despite therapy, he didn't improve, and after months he decided to end his life by stopping his tube feedings.

My spirit constantly wanted to be free. Would it have been a sin to set it free? I don't know, but I do know that I would have chosen death rather than live like that. I expect I wouldn't have waited twelve months with no improvement before I asked for the tube feedings to stop.

Jill later told me that I wasn't crying that morning when I asked her about assisted suicide, even though my emotions were quite labile (meaning my emotions were unpredictable and beyond my ability to control, as a result of the brainstem damage). She looked away, quietly crying, and said, "Yes."

I could tell she didn't mean it. She had said *yes* just to shut me up. I realized it was too much for her to comprehend. She needed time to think. This was just the first step. But I was serious; I needed to know I had the option of ending my life. I had to end the discussion then and broach the subject slowly, in small increments, to give us both time to think. I felt so sorry for Jill.

I never did talk to her again about allowing me to die, because I started to improve. Before I left the Saint John Regional Hospital, my left thumb and neck had started to move a little. Now, at Stan Cassidy, these movements improved, along with new movements in my fingers and arms. I expected this rate of recovery to continue. I was still locked in — none of the movements were functional — but I replaced hopelessness with hope.

I needed hope. I reacted to any small new movement with an excitement disproportionate to the change. I had hope of walking again, hope of using my arms, hope of speaking.

Looking back, twenty years later, I see how important hope was and still is to me. Without hope there is the danger of giving up and then it is almost guaranteed there will be no improvement. Hope is healthy as long as we're willing to accept reality when all attempts have failed.

June was a month of emotions as I settled into Stan Cassidy and got used to the idea of being a disabled person. Father's

Day was especially difficult. I couldn't stop the tears when my children presented me with gifts. They had made me cards that said the sweetest things. They knew my emotions were fragile, so they didn't lay it on too thick. I felt bad for them when I cried. It must be traumatic for children to see their dad cry. But Jill had prepared them well. She had explained to them that I really couldn't help crying; it was a side effect of the stroke. My children seemed to be able to accept my tears with smiles and hugs and avoided crying in response. I had Jill to thank for this, as I do for so many things.

Colin, our twenty-year-old son, brought my dog up to see me. Jenny was an eight-year-old miniature German schnauzer. I was quite fond of her, and there was no doubt who her master was. I groomed her, took her for walks, and played with her, and I was usually the one who fed her. We had a favourite route for our walks and a special area where I let her off the leash so she could go into the woods to poop and then come back. I found these walks enjoyable, therapeutic, and a way to unwind from a busy day.

Now I was afraid to see her. I envisaged a scene: Jenny would jump for joy at seeing me and I would cry in front of everyone. Jenny would be jumping up on my lap, licking my face, glad to have me back. People standing around in front of Stan Cassidy would see this grown man crying over a little dog.

I needn't have worried. Colin parked on the far side of the parking lot so I could be away from people. Colin lifted Jenny from the truck and let her explore the lawn. By this time, I had gained some ability to use a power wheelchair independently by left-arm control, so I slowly motored across the lot toward her. Jenny stopped sniffing the grass and watched me approach. She didn't jump for joy, run to me, or even wag her tail. She looked at me and then through me. Her eyes glazed over and she resumed sniffing the ground, occasionally greeting Jill or our kids, but pretending I didn't exist.

In a curious way, it was a relief. It spared me the pain and tears that a joyful greeting would have brought. It made it easier to say goodbye when it was time for her to leave. I still cried; in fact, I cried in anticipation before I even saw her.

I understood when her eyes glazed over. Months before my stroke, I had read *The Hidden Life of Dogs* by Elizabeth Marshall Thomas. She described how domesticated dogs retain a fair amount of their natural wild-pack-dog behaviour. When left on their own, a group of domestic dogs quickly revert to the social behaviour of wild pack dogs. They have a leader — the alpha — whom they all obey. She surmised that a solitary dog treats its human family like a pack. Someone becomes the alpha, the leader it obeys and respects. Dogs do not want to be the alpha, but they will assume the role if need be. This is why you need to be firm but loving with your dog; if a dog assumes the role of alpha, watch out!

I expect I was the alpha in Jenny's world. An alpha wolf has the responsibility, at the very least, to be around to protect the pack. If the alpha is disgraced by another wolf or by not doing his duties, he is ostracized by the pack. He is "not seen" by the others; he becomes a lone wolf. In Jenny's eyes, by suddenly vanishing from the family and turning up here at Stan Cassidy, I was a disgrace. I had gone from alpha to lone wolf, as she expressed by not seeing me or affording me any welcome.

This I understood. There was no doubt she knew who I was; her sense of smell was keen. Yet I was in a wheelchair, a contraption she had never seen. I was breathing through a tube in my throat, and I made no sound to greet her. I didn't pat her, play with her, or use my arms. I didn't even smile. How was she to react? It was all too confusing to her, so she reacted in the only way she knew: she ignored the whole situation. She pretended I didn't even exist until she could make some sense of it.

I don't know if Jenny's reaction was a normal canine social reaction or confusion or a combination of both, but when I wrote the first edition of this book, two years after my stroke, she was just then warming up to me. Jill had supplanted me as her alpha. Jenny accepted the wheelchair but she didn't like it. She either didn't understand or refused to recognize my voice, probably because I sounded gruff, with little variation in pitch. I didn't mind — it was nice just to be accepted back into her pack.

As I've already mentioned, my emotions were hard to control. I cried over everything: letters, cards, friends, Jill's leaving, Jill's arriving. It didn't matter what it was; I cried. I felt embarrassed when I cried in front of people.

In one incident, I cried in front of an assembly of staff. Two patients, Dwight and Eric, had been at the centre for a long time. They had progressed to the point where they were being discharged. All the staff and patients gathered in a big circle in the cafeteria. When the farewell speeches were made, I burst into tears. Luckily, I couldn't make a sound, but I was ashamed of the tears streaming down my face.

Another time, my mom and stepfather decided it would be good for me to get out of Stan Cassidy for a while. They had brought a war movie with them from Saint John and we went over to Kiwanis House to watch it. I cried seeing men being killed. Crying over a war movie!

I knew the staff members were used to emotional lability in post-stroke patients, and I was used to it in my own practice, but experiencing it myself was difficult. I was the doctor. I was the one who helped people through tragedies and death. I didn't cry. In fact, before my stroke, I hadn't cried in years. I knew it was foolish to think this way, but I couldn't help feeling that I looked weak.

The emotional turmoil eased gradually over many months. It was a relief to finally gain control. For me, these exaggerated emotions were perhaps the worst thing about my stroke. Foolish pride!

I wish I could cry now. It was a good release. A good cry would feel better than anger and frustration.

I cried whenever Jill had to leave for Saint John. I knew she had to go. She had business to attend to, our children needed her, and besides, she had nowhere to stay when the Kiwanis was full, as it often was. It didn't matter; I cried when I knew she had to leave. My mom and stepfather tried to fill the void by staying nearby when Jill was absent.

I'm ashamed because I know I made it harder for Jill to leave me. It was tough for her to see me cry, and if she could only have seen me a few minutes later, she would have known I was fine. My friend Barbie often came in to sit with me and we would watch reruns of *Seinfeld*.

Jill was afraid I might need someone but not be able to ring the bell. I could move my left thumb, so when she left, she would place the call bell in my left hand so I could buzz for attention if I needed to.

There is one night I am especially ashamed of. It was a Sunday evening. The kids had spent the weekend at our cottage. My parents have a cottage close to ours, so I knew the kids were fine and enjoying themselves. My children later told me that they liked the responsibility of looking after the cottage. I think they appreciated the fact that we trusted them. Jill, who had been with me, was heading home for a few days. The day had been sunny. Normally, I would have been heading back to the city after spending a weekend at the cottage, but the reality was I was here at Stan Cassidy. I wished so much to be going home with Jill. I suddenly missed my kids, the cottage, driving, the freedom to do what I wanted. I felt trapped. I wanted out — anywhere but here. *It's not fair!* As Jill, with tears in her eyes, was about to leave, I made matters worse by motioning with my left arm that I wanted to slash my wrist. I was angry, but tears were streaming down my face. I felt I had no control of my body, my desires, or my emotions. I wanted Jill to feel my pain.

I am so ashamed of my irrational actions when I think of them now. Jill hated to leave me and I compounded the problem. I eventually got hold of myself and tried to stop crying by immersing myself in a TV program. I realized I was acting foolish, but I was still angry. We talked it out like always, except this time I had to communicate slowly and incompletely through the eye-gaze board. Still, once I was able to "verbalize" my feelings, I felt relief.

After a while, Barbie came in to keep me company. The tears were gone and I enjoyed her conversation. When she left, I continued to stare at the TV, not aware of what was on, thinking of what had just occurred, of life, and feeling sorry for myself. Soon the nurses came in to prepare me for bed and gave me that sweet sleeping pill, which I welcomed, so that I could slip away and stop thinking.

Most stroke survivors feel anger at some point. You can be accepting for only so long. Eventually, the frustration or a feeling of unfairness boils over. You have been wronged and someone is going to hear about it! Unfortunately, it is often the one you love. Many marriages break up after a stroke. Some people never get over their anger and constantly blame their spouse for being well.

I fought the anger by realizing that nobody owed me anything. I had a choice: engage in self-pity and anger or move on.

Channel that energy wasted on anger to physical exertion, Shawn, I thought. *Remember, bad things happen — they just do. Get over it and move on.*

I have the advantage of being a family doctor, so I have been involved in counselling post-stroke victims and families. However, anger still crept into me. I suppose it was okay. I let it happen, I dealt with it, and I moved on. I tried to remind myself that Jill was not to blame for being well and she had a life to live. *Don't begrudge her that,* I told myself.

I also had experience with being ashamed; I had once acted so unprofessionally.

CHAPTER 12
SAMANTHA

Samantha went to school with me from grades one to twelve. We didn't live close together, so she was never a playmate of mine, but we had a friendly, respectful, comfortable relationship. I hadn't seen her in nearly twenty years when one day my receptionist told me she had just taken a call from an old friend of mine who would like to speak to me.

I was delighted to call Samantha back at the end of the day, and after a short conversation to reconnect, she told me the reason for the call: her family physician had either left town or discharged her from his practice, or she felt he wasn't helping her. I have forgotten what the reason was, but she needed a doctor. She asked if I could help her.

I felt sorry for Samantha after she conveyed her concerns about her health. I could feel her pain and desperation. I paused. Looking after friends can be difficult for a physician, but I'd had no contact with Samantha in twenty years. Surely there would be no lingering effects after that length of time. I was sure I could act and advise her like a professional. I was confident in my abilities as a doctor. I needed to help her and agreed to see her the next week.

After my first appointment with her, I felt the most likely diagnosis was chronic fatigue syndrome, but this is a diagnosis made only by ruling out other potential problems. I ordered a number of tests and reviewed her past results.

I saw her every week or two over the next several months. Conventional medicine had no cure to offer, just supportive therapy that included medication and psychotherapy. I, along with the other doctors she had seen, could be wrong, so it was imperative to keep an open mind and search for another possible diagnosis. Besides, perhaps medicine had just not found the cause of this malady yet. Today, for example, before making a diagnosis, I would rule out Lyme disease, which back then wasn't on our radar as a possible cause of chronic fatigue.

Samantha was very intent on a cure, as anyone would be, and didn't accept the diagnosis of chronic fatigue syndrome. I readily agreed to send her to specialists to rule out diseases we might have overlooked, but after months of consultations with multiple doctors, it was time to start accepting and work intently with the diagnosis we had. It is well known that people who don't accept a diagnosis or who continue to search for a magical cure are more likely to do poorly. The mind is a powerful tool in maintaining good health. Accepting a working diagnosis would not have to mean abandoning hope in the search for another cause of her fatigue.

After she had seen a third specialist, I thought I'd introduce the possibility of psychotherapy to help her deal with the symptoms, as well as trying some complementary alternative medical therapies, as long as they were safe and inexpensive. I had softly planted the idea of trying other things if the therapies I was using were not helping, but Samantha had other ideas. She wanted to go to a major clinic in the United States for assessment.

I was getting frustrated. All patients have the right to deal with their health in any way they want, within reason, even if I don't agree. But it is my duty in a socialized medical system to try to minimize financial burden to the health system by not ordering needless tests or consultations. Normally by now, in a situation like Samantha's, I would have voiced my skepticism of seeing a certain specialist or doing another test. If the patient truly wanted that consult or test, I wouldn't have refused, but I would have given my opinion of the futility of the venture. Now, by not expressing my professional opinion, I was getting frustrated.

Was it because Samantha was an old friend? In general, people don't like to be too critical of friends and they try to accept different ways, views, and mannerisms. Perhaps the bond I had forged with Samantha over those years of childhood and into our teens was suppressing my professional demeanour. In any case, I didn't say much that I can remember about her planned trip for another opinion, and I helped her by writing letters, copying test results, and obtaining copies of X-rays to take with her.

Samantha and her husband, Gary, came to see me one afternoon after their return. I had received a summary from the clinic in the United States earlier that week, and unsurprisingly, they hadn't changed the working diagnosis or shed light on any other avenue of investigation. It was late Friday afternoon when Samantha and Gary came to my office. In fact, my receptionist had left for the day and Samantha was my last patient. It had been a long, trying day. I was very tired.

Gary came in to the examination room with Samantha, which was unusual, and before I said a word about the results of the assessment, he said, "What other doctor can she see?"

I exploded. In a loud voice I asked Gary what he thought *I* was. Was I just a means to get to *real* doctors? Did my opinion count for nothing? I went on. I stood up like I was challenging him physically. Samantha stood up and tried to calm me down, telling Gary to leave the examination room, which he did. For the rest of the appointment, Samantha and I didn't talk much about the clinic visit. Instead, I spent most of the time telling her that I couldn't be her doctor, but that I would find her a good one and that it was for the best.

After the weekend, I asked a colleague of mine, who I felt was one of the best family physicians in the city, if she would take Samantha as her patient. I explained the conflict I was having looking after her — patient versus friend — but not the details of our Friday appointment, and she kindly offered to take over her care. I never saw Samantha again.

My conduct at that last visit was very unprofessional. I never spoke to any patient, before or since, in that manner. It was inexcusable behaviour for a physician or any other professional. I had let a smouldering, unexpressed emotion erupt at the first suspected slight of my abilities as a doctor. The truth is Samantha and Gary probably never even entertained the idea that I was incompetent, even unconsciously. The notion was all in my head.

Gary didn't deserve my wrath. He was asking a simple question with no disrespect intended. In fact, he might have been trying to gently convey to his wife that further investigation was futile. Gary might have been a support for me in helping Samantha.

I was tired. It had been a long day and week. If I remember correctly, I'd had to tell someone bad news a few hours earlier. But none of that excuses me for my unprofessional behaviour. I would have apologized to both of them by now, but I have forgotten her married name.

I imagine we all have done or said something in our lives that we wish we could take back. Sometimes we can apologize, redo, or compensate to make amends, and sometimes we can't — what's done is done.

I cringe when I think of my behaviour that late afternoon, and I should never forget, but I have forgiven myself. I am only human and subject to all the frailties of being imperfect. I can try to do my very best, but I will never be perfect. I had to forgive myself.

I also forgave myself for being angry at Jill that she could leave the rehabilitation centre without me, for showing her I wanted to kill myself, for making her cry. I had poor control of my emotions at the time, and I was in the anger stage of loss. I do forgive myself, but that doesn't stop me from sadly remembering the moments I hurt Jill.

I knew Jill had forgiven me the moment I saw her when she returned to Stan Cassidy Centre a few days later. July was upon us.

CHAPTER 13
EARLY JULY

Near the end of June, a colleague from home visited me and told me the Saint John Medical Society had raised money for my family by holding a dinner dance. He was on his way to rent an apartment for Jill and my family to stay in while in Fredericton.

I was floored by this gesture of generosity and love from my colleagues. I felt I didn't deserve it. If I could have talked, I would have stumbled over words of thanks, but also words of refusal: *This is way too much. We're okay. Donate the money,* and other excuses why we should not accept the gift. I found it hard to accept such generosity without returning the favour in some way. I would receive many such gifts and acts of love over the next few months, and I learned to accept them with humility and love. I learned people want to be kind and loving, without any expectations. Giving and loving freely have their own rewards. I learned to accept with that same love.

Having Jill nearby was a blessing. I didn't have to worry about her driving from Saint John, and it boosted my spirits when she arrived at physiotherapy each morning.

In July, the heat continued. I was usually decked out in a T-shirt, shorts, sneakers, and, of course, my beautiful white antiembolic stockings. I was still in my private room because of my trach care, my tube feedings, and the high-level nursing care I required.

I got out more now because I had graduated to a power chair (the word *electric* has undesirable connotations when discussing chairs). I couldn't use my left hand, but I could move my arm a bit from my shoulder. Doreen, my occupational therapist, strapped my forearm into an armrest that controlled the chair. To make it go forward, I pressed down; up for backward; into my body to go right; and away for turning left. The outward motion of my forearm was the hardest for me to make, and still is. Both of my arms preferred to stay curled up against my body and protested any attempt to move them otherwise.

I spent many hours going around in circles. If I relaxed for a second, my arm tone brought the control in and I would start to go right, around and around, until I managed to relax that limb (after a stroke, some muscles are missing the signal to relax, leaving the muscle with a high resting tone that is hard to break). To spare the walls of Stan Cassidy, I practised manoeuvring my chair in the parking lot.

I had to be placed in my seat like an astronaut. And in fact, it did take a team of nurses to accomplish this task, but I was most grateful, for finally I had some freedom. Before I got the power wheelchair, I had been dependent on the nursing staff or Jill for transportation. Now I felt independent, being able to read the schedule board in the hallway, which listed each patient's name, the days of the week, and the schedule for each type of therapy, and then head down to my therapy sessions on my own. When I wanted to go for a breath of fresh air, I could go out the automatic main doors by myself. Fresh air! What a treat. I couldn't thank Doreen enough for this newfound freedom.

I saw fellow patients more. To say I *interacted* with them would not be quite right; mostly, I eavesdropped upon their conversations. There were wide assortments of injuries, diseases, and ages. I looked quite a sight, but I didn't feel too out of place among this lot. We limped, wheeled, swore inappropriately, laughed, and cried; we did it all.

We were all facing major changes in our lives — some more than others — but the attitude that prevailed in Stan Cassidy was positive. It could have been a sad place, a place of broken lives, but instead there was hope and love. Don't get the wrong impression; there was tragedy, frustration, tears, broken hearts, and anger, but the staff never let the mood become sombre.

I enjoyed being with my fellow patients. I listened, laughed by coughing gobs of phlegm out my trach at some joke, and then usually ended my "conversation" by farting. Oh, I was quite the social butterfly!

It was so hard to converse. By the time I spelled out a joke to Jill about something someone had said, the conversation had moved on to another topic and my joke was received with puzzlement. Never try to tell a joke with an eye-gaze board.

I was never shunned. My fellow patients always made room for me. I tried my best to turn away when I laughed so they didn't get a gob of phlegm flying their way. They didn't know it, but I talked with them the whole time. I thought I was very funny.

I wanted very much to talk with my fellow patients. After all, misery loves company. I wanted to ask them and tell them things that only other patients would understand. *How is your day going? I feel miserable. I couldn't lift my left hand up to my chest today. I did that yesterday. Mereille is so nice to me. How's Carly to work with? Isn't it a pain to have to go to bed so early! How are you sleeping, by the way?*

I would have enjoyed commiserating with someone, sharing feelings. By being locked in, I was locked out. I was alone with my thoughts and feelings. Thank God I had Jill. I communicated through her to my fellow patients. I was a patient first, not a doctor, and I needed their camaraderie.

I wanted to discuss feelings with someone besides Jill. How were they coping? Did they have bad days, too? Jill got it all, and even at that it was superficial because of my difficulties communicating. I gained a new appreciation for people who are deaf or cannot speak, and the problems they must encounter. If you are locked out, I hope you have someone who knows that you are still in there and need to communicate.

We are social animals; communication in some form is essential. I missed it — big time! Even to be able to wave hello, nod, or smile in passing would have been a relief. Having a coffee, talking about the weather, engaging in small talk within a group — how I longed for interaction!

I am a quiet fellow; always have been and, especially now, always will be. It is perhaps appropriate that I should experience this malady. I was shy growing up, and later, when I grew out of my shyness, others always seemed to say things better than I could. I made up for this quietness at home. I joked, played my guitar, sang, and talked all the time. My children's impression of me is probably far different than that of my colleagues. Until I had my stroke, I don't think I appreciated how devastating the effects of aphasic, or speech problems were in stroke victims, how isolating and lonely they are.

My socialization was fair, using Jill as my go-between, but communicating with the nursing staff continued to be tedious. Most had little knowledge of the eye-gaze board, and they continued to point to each letter rather than watching where my gaze was. I felt perhaps they could have held a session to instruct the staff on how to communicate with me. The eye-gaze board was simple and fast to learn. I had to give the nurses credit, though: no matter how busy they were, most tried to understand what I was saying.

Doreen and Beth explored all manner of communicative devices with me. They chose them depending on my ability at the time. For example, when I regained movement in my neck so that I could move my head from side to side, big button-type buzzers were hung on either side of my headrest. I was supposed to learn Morse code and then, through a computer, I would be able to communicate.

Thankfully, I moved beyond this point of ability within two weeks, as my left hand improved. I then attempted a similar Morse code method with my hand. I tried one weekend to learn Morse code, but my heart wasn't in it. *As soon as they get this trach out, I'm going to talk*, I told myself. *Damn it! What is the point of wasting so much energy learning Morse code?*

They were trying to use whatever ability I had at any given moment in a functional way. I knew that. Yet I balked. Doreen put a device on my forehead that moved a cursor on a computer. I thought it was very interesting but also very disheartening. *I won't need this*, I thought. *I'm improving far beyond needing a laser stuck to my forehead!*

I was scared they thought this was as far as I'd get. I tried to be a good patient and act interested, but really I was thinking, *No way, José! These instruments are for disabled people!*

Disability was hard to accept. Inside, I felt the same. I didn't feel disabled. Besides, some people were telling me my condition would continue to improve. Yes, but there has to be a time when we say, "Well, I guess that's it!" Doesn't there?

I would accept my current abilities, or try to, and move on. There is a difference between acceptance and giving up. Just because I accept that I won't walk doesn't mean I have abandoned all hope that someday I will walk. These questions tormented me: Does the acceptance of reality stop possible progression? If I doubt my ability to walk, will it prevent me from obtaining that goal? If I say, "I *will* walk," does it increase my chances?

It was hard to always fail in physiotherapy. I couldn't do very much. Mereille asked me to sit on the side of the exercise cot. Betty, the physio assistant, and Mereille manipulated me into a sitting position, my spine bent forward like the Hunchback of Notre Dame. I was expending a huge amount of energy just trying to keep my head up, and my legs were giving me no support as I swayed with Mereille and Betty on either side.

"Straighten your back, Shawn," Mereille said.

I barely perceived a movement.

"Gooda!" she exclaimed in her francophone dialect.

I let out a whoosh-squeak through my trach. I had barely perceived a movement, but Mereille had said it was "gooda"!

This scene repeated itself throughout my stay: Mereille would say "gooda" at some small achievement and I would laugh. I'm glad they thought it was laughter, because sometimes it was a cry. When I achieved some small goal, I felt like crying for joy. I felt like crying for bending back my left wrist another inch, for bending my knee, for many small movements. I was so desperate for any improvement, any sign that I was becoming "normal." *Let them think I'm laughing at Mereille's exuberance,* I thought. *It's less embarrassing this way.*

The gymnasium where physio took place was huge, with two big rooms. Unlike the rest of the centre, it was modern and had the best of equipment. There were bright colours, lots of windows, and many smiles. Energy circulated around the room with the whirl of machines, shouted encouragements, and pockets of laughter.

Mereille chose a cot with a blue mat that had a steel mesh platform over it. It would be my mat for the next ten months. It was electronic; they could raise or lower it by foot pedals. A poster on the wall, next to the mat, of whales swimming in a bay became my focus for tranquility.

I eventually did master some semblance of sitting without looking like a hunchback. The nursing staff had been using a Hoyer lift to transfer me from my bed to my wheelchair and back, but now I had enough body strength to progress to a sliding board. The Hoyer lift is a powered device used to transfer patients without manually lifting them. The sensation of swinging through the air is exactly like the feeling you get on a swing. I did not like the sensation in the least. I never complained — after all, what could they do? — but there did seem to be nurses who delighted in giving me an extra spin. I was scared of heights as it was, and this experience did nothing to alleviate my fear. In fact, my phobia seemed to get worse; during this period, I would get a peculiar sensation in the pit of my stomach whenever a high-angle shot was shown on TV.

When I graduated from bed baths to tub baths, I was brought to the bathroom on the Hoyer lift, perched precariously like a baby in a stork's beak, down the corridor, stark naked, all the while trying to smile. I was covered by a blanket, but I knew, and anyone I met along the way knew, that I was naked underneath. It was hard to keep up appearances while dangling in the air, naked.

The bathroom was just big enough for the tub and a nurse on each side, and no more. It was a tricky manoeuvre to get the Hoyer lift and me through the narrow doorway and into the bath, all the while preserving my dignity. Once I was in the bath, the nurses scrubbed me furiously from either side. I was completely at their mercy. My trach was just above the waterline, while my arms and legs floated uselessly just below the surface.

The tub had a whirlpool feature that I couldn't use because of my trach. The nurses forgot once and turned on the whirlpool. The water rose and bubbled dangerously close to my open trach. I fluttered my eyelids furiously to warn them, expecting to aspirate water at any moment. The nurses quickly turned off the whirlpool action when they realized their mistake, but not before I had transformed into a human board, my body in a massive total spasm from the stress.

After the bath, I took another ride on the Hoyer lift to dry off in my room. So I was Hoyered in and out of bed, onto my exercise mat and off, and into and out of my bath. When I entertained the thought of writing an account of my journey, I thought I might call it *Life on the Hoyer Lift*, in the vein of Mark Twain's *Life on the Mississippi*.

I had to find some humour in my life; otherwise it was pretty sad. The Hoyer lift reminded me of how dependent I had become on machines and people to do just the simplest of tasks. Luckily, under Mereille and Doreen's guidance, I graduated to the sliding board. This is simply a highly polished board that bridges the gap between two objects so a patient can slide across. Some people learn to do this independently, but not me! I was no star at this, either. I didn't have enough mobility in my trunk or enough strength in my arms, and maybe I had too much lead in my bottom, to accomplish this. In the months I used this technique, I always needed people to help me slide along.

The sliding board enabled me to enjoy another activity: going for a car ride. Doreen took me for a short ride soon after I came to the centre, but I was hardly able to keep my head up, so I hadn't enjoyed the experience. Now that I had better head control, I was eager to try again.

Charlie was an assistant in occupational therapy who loved to joke around. He told us his alter persona was named Charlene, because he was pretty handy with a sewing machine. Charlie always had a humorous story to tell. He was a perfect employee for Stan Cassidy. I wished I could have laughed instead of spitting at him!

Charlie took Jill and me for my first long car ride. I did all right — at least I got through it without needing to have my trach suctioned. However, the trip did make me nauseated, but I didn't tell them. I had reasons for keeping quiet.

I wanted to go home. The weekends were driving me crazy. I mourned what I had lost, and by this time, I *knew* I had lost them. I used to love getting up early on Saturday morning, making my rounds at the hospital, and then coming back home to start my chores. I loved working around our home and cottage. Completing tasks gave me a sense of accomplishment.

At Stan Cassidy, I continued to wake up early, and one Saturday before our car ride I woke up to a glorious sunny day. It was about five thirty and the room was already heating up from the sun pouring in the windows. The air conditioner had been on all night, but it was unable to keep up with the sun's heat. I became hot and uncomfortable and struggled to trigger the call bell beside my head. When I finally succeeded in signalling the nurse, she opened the window wider for me and turned on the TV on the way out.

I was not interested in what was on and I didn't have the ability to change the channel. But I needed some relief from my thoughts. Normally, I'd be at the cottage. *Let's see, what needs to be done?* I thought. *The deck needs stain in a few areas. Got to plant those new plants I purchased. Got to fix that bank by the back of the house. Boat needs a good scrubbing. Wait! I can't do these things! I will never be able to do these things!* I tortured myself with negative thoughts. I wanted so desperately to do something with my hands to take my mind off everything. *Get up! Get busy!*

An hour went by, then two hours. A nurse came in to start my tube feeding. *Great, I'll be here another two hours!* Think, think, think! That was all I could do. Jill was at home. I didn't have her to talk to. I didn't think of it then, but I should have had an audiobook available for those times.

I had now been awake for four hours. I wanted to do something. I wanted to move, to stop thinking, to feel the air. I wanted to swing my legs out of this bed and walk! I got frustrated. I grew angry with everyone. *No one knows what this is like!*

The nurses stopped my tube feeding and told me they would be back. I waited another hour. Thinking, thinking. The cartoons on TV irritated me and made me sad because I had no way to turn them off. I was reduced to watching them on a Saturday morning instead of being out in the sun. I was so frustrated, I felt like screaming. I wanted to get up. I felt trapped.

When a nurse finally did return, she began to bathe me and prepare me for the day. I started to cry. I had cried before over silly things like a war movie, but this was the first time I had ever shared my frustrations over my condition with anyone other than Jill. The nurse showed empathy and explained that she had thought she was doing me a favour by letting me sleep in on a Saturday morning.

I couldn't stay mad at her, but when she placed me outside the front door, I remained depressed. The day was beautiful and I couldn't enjoy it. I had wasted more than five hours doing nothing. I felt hurt; this wasn't fair! *I don't deserve this! I've always been kind,* I reasoned. *I never intentionally hurt anyone. I help others. I've tried to be a good Christian. I loved God and my neighbour. I wanted to grow old, see grandchildren, bounce them on my knee, throw them up in the air, make them laugh. Now they'll see this figure who can't hold them and doesn't smile. Hard to love that! Why? Why? Why?*

A while later, my parents arrived and found me sitting outside in a dark mood. I told them through the eye-gaze board how frustrated I was from the morning. I did not tell them how depressed I felt. I knew that would make them feel terrible and sad. Besides, I just didn't want to talk about it. I felt better by the afternoon, probably from the social interaction.

That morning made me determined to leave Stan Cassidy on the weekends. *If I could only get home for two days*, I thought, *I could tolerate five days here.*

So that was why I didn't tell Charlie and Jill that the car ride had made me nauseated. I had started to plan and to get Jill used to the idea of bringing me home for the weekends. Naturally, she was afraid of the responsibility of my care. There was my trach care, tube feedings, transfers, turning during the night, and a lot of other things to consider.

Jill accepted the challenge because she knew how desperately I wanted to leave on the weekends. I can never thank her enough. It didn't surprise me that she was willing to try. She was a nurse, and this greatly facilitated her learning process. The nurses showed her how to suction my trach, keep it clean, use the infusion pump for my feeds, and transfer me.

I wanted Jill to express her concerns, but I knew she might be reluctant to in case it appeared she didn't want me home. It was important for me to really listen and not discount her fears in my enthusiasm to get home for the weekends. Many years before, I had learned to actively listen to what people were saying.

CHAPTER 14
STEVE

Great lessons are learned in the practice of medicine. I learned from almost every encounter dealing with human life, emotions, and tragedies. Some of these lessons were painful. One of my most painful lessons involved Steve.

Steve owned his own business and was moderately successful. I saw him often because he had hypertension, or high blood pressure, that was hard to control, as well as insomnia. His insomnia was the worst case I had ever encountered. I tried the entire selection of regular non-pharmaceutical remedies, all the hypnotics, mild tranquilizers, psychological methods — everything. Although he didn't seem depressed, I thought he might have an atypical or masked case of depression, so we tried antidepressants. I referred him to psychiatrists, psychologists, neurologists, and any other specialty I could think of, however remote the possibility that it would make a difference. Nothing helped!

Those were the days before the advent of sleep labs. We were not yet aware of sleep apnea and the role it plays in our general health. Steve would have been an ideal candidate for a sleep study, and constant positive airway pressure, now used to treat sleep apnea, could perhaps have been his cure. We'll never know.

Somehow, Steve maintained a good sense of humour throughout his ordeal, and we had a good doctor-patient relationship. One day, he came into the office with a sore ankle. X-rays and blood work revealed nothing. It got worse despite anti-inflammatory drugs, used to treat arthritis, and local treatments, such as applying heat and cold. A bone scan of his ankle revealed nothing. I was perplexed but not worried — he had no other symptoms — and I sent him to a rheumatoid specialist. In the meantime, I was going on vacation. A locum tenens, a doctor who takes over a practice for a short period, would see my patients while I was gone.

I had a great time on my vacation, until the final week. My locum phoned me with bad news that she felt I would want to know. Steve had been admitted to hospital, and he had widespread cancer. Apparently, he had gone to the ER with bad chest pain. The X-ray was suspicious, and a total bone scan confirmed that he had widespread cancer in his bones. Hardly any area had been spared; it was most unusual. The news hit me right in the stomach. I was numb.

I struggled through the rest of my vacation, trying to act happy for the family, but my mind was elsewhere. I had trouble sleeping, as I pored over each office visit in my mind. What had I missed? I had done a localized bone scan because it was cheaper and I could get it faster. If only I had done a total scan! After going over everything, I was convinced I had not missed anything. Steve had never complained of any other pain or symptoms. Besides, the ankle pain was probably metastasis — cancer that had spread — so it would likely have been too late by then, anyway. But why hadn't my X-rays and localized bone scan shown anything?

I tormented myself with self-doubts. I knew that regardless of whether I had or had not done a good job, in the eyes of a layperson it looked as though I had completely misdiagnosed Steve's condition. I suppose I had, but with the information I was presented with, I had done my best.

I couldn't take it anymore. I had to see Steve. I left my family at the cottage and drove to the hospital.

His wife was not my patient. She did not know me. I anticipated that she would be angry and suspicious of me. I used to feel hurt when people showed their anger toward me when a loved one was dying. But I grew to realize that anger is a normal stage of grieving. Doctors have to learn to accept or understand the anger directed toward them, even if it is inappropriate. If people can be angry with God over a loved one's death, it should not be surprising that they might be angry with the doctor.

Steve's wife was more composed than I expected. She was a little confrontational, but who wouldn't be? I was anxious about this meeting and about seeing Steve, so I wasn't really listening when she said, "Whatever you do, don't tell him what he's got!"

I heard, but I didn't hear. I was moving into his room and just nodded. After I had greeted Steve, I asked him to tell me what had happened, how his symptoms were, how they were treating him in the hospital. He got out of bed and sat in a chair beside me.

He stared into my eyes and asked, "What's wrong with me?" I realized with horror what his wife had just said and what I had agreed to by nodding. I had never lied to a patient before. Most of the literature on death and dying states that you should be open and frank with a dying patient. The unknown is more frightening than knowing. I have always tried to answer patients' questions truthfully, while leaving them with some hope. I don't give them bleak forecasts, even if the outlook is dire, unless asked.

That moment is forever frozen in time for me, like the little girl's face in the truck I had nearly hit that had got me into this mess. I felt Steve's wife glaring at me from behind him. I felt Steve's eyes searching my face, imploring me for the truth. I told him.

That scene plays over and over in my mind. It has been more than twenty years since Steve died and I still wonder whether I was right to tell him. I've concluded no. I handled the whole situation poorly.

Every dying patient has the right to know, and Steve's eyes seemed to be saying that he was frantic for the truth. I think someone should have told him, but not me. I went against his wife's wishes when I should have respected them. When she told me her wish that I not tell him his diagnosis, I should have listened and then taken the time to explain my position. If she didn't agree with my belief that the dying have the right to know the truth if they ask, I should have never gone into the room.

Because I wasn't the attending physician, I could have told him, "I can't answer that. You'll have to ask the doctor who's treating you here." But that smelled like a cop-out to me. I have heard too many pass-the-buck answers in hospitals. A patient can leave hospital not knowing exactly what transpired. However, in this instance, if I had wanted to continue to see Steve and abide with his wife's request not to tell him, avoiding a true response might have been the best option.

I was wrong. I learned to always — no matter how tired I was, how rushed, how bored — listen to what was being said to me. Not only by patients: by anyone.

Steve's autopsy did not reveal the primary tumour. His body was riddled with adenocarcinoma but they were all small metastases. I spoke to the pathologist, and he assured me he had looked everywhere carefully. I suspect the primary site might have been the kidney. No matter where the primary site was, it must have been very small, probably too small to cause symptoms for an early detection and cure.

It's very unusual for a small tumour to spread so widely in the body. Something was drastically wrong with Steve's immune system. Sleep is needed for the body to repair itself. I have often wondered if Steve's immune system was compromised because of his terrible insomnia.

CHAPTER 15
LATE JULY

Planning for coming home on the weekends made me happy and excited. Finally, an active, positive, exciting venture to look forward to. Patti, a friend of ours, arranged the nursing schedule at home. I needed nurses at night for safety, to turn me every two hours, and to clean my trach. Jill couldn't possibly do all of this twenty-four hours a day.

The nurses at Stan Cassidy encouraged us and tried to allay any fears Jill might have. I was not the least bit afraid; I had complete confidence in Jill. I understood the pressure she must feel over having me at home alone, all the scenarios that could happen, but I needed to go home. I was lucky that I had a wife who was a nurse and there was room in our home for a rented hospital bed, an infusion pump, and a suction machine. Plus I had insurance that covered nursing help.

We had lists of all the paraphernalia we would need: infusion pump, suction catheters, condom catheters, cans of tube feed, incontinence pads, and much more. The centre loaned us the infusion pump and suction machine. Finally, after weeks of planning, we were ready.

Our little car was loaded down. Louise, the head nurse, and Karen, an occupational therapist who took over my care during Doreen's vacation, followed us with even more equipment. Meanwhile, I looked like a dead man wearing sunglasses, sitting in a car going for a ride. My face was frozen, and I was propped upright in the passenger seat with pillows on either side of my body. It amused me to think of what I must look like to other drivers, something out of a horror story or a comedy.

The nurses were afraid I might need suctioning in the car, so we took an emergency portable suction along with us. Luckily, I didn't need it.

The trip from Fredericton to Saint John passes through a huge army training ground, Canadian Forces Base Gagetown, and miles of uninhabited forest. It felt so normal to be in a car, watching the scenery as we passed by, but also exciting after two months of institutionalization.

I felt like a kid returning home after a prolonged summer vacation. It felt surreal to be somewhere so familiar. I was the outcast here. The lawn, the tree beside the driveway, the front deck were all as they had been. It was I who had changed. I was the surreal one.

Jill had had a ramp built around the side of our home onto the back deck so I could get into our house. When she wheeled me onto the deck, I saw that some of our friends had decorated the railings with balloons and welcome-home signs. A lump grew in my throat, and as I entered the back door and saw the round, two-sided fireplace that was the focal point of our home, my tears started. I felt foolish in front of Karen and Louise, but for the first time I had some control in preventing an all-out bawling. Karen and Louise quickly got things in place, assessed that I would be safe, and left.

Alone — for the first time in more than two months, there were no nurses or doctors around. I was quietly ecstatic. The first place I asked Jill to take me was outside on our deck, but it was cloudy and foggy, so I didn't spend very long there. Later, as Jill wheeled me by the stairs, I longingly glanced up toward our bedroom, wishing I could seek comfort in my own bed. I expected to be able to ascend those stairs one of these days, at first by going up backward on my behind, using my arms to lift me up step by step. My left arm was improving, and I expected my right arm to follow suit.

Jill had rented a hospital bed for me and set it up in our living room. I eventually rested in bed and had my tube feeding. The kids arrived home from school, and a few of my friends visited. The company over the next few weekends was steady, maybe tiring, but a good thing; they kept me from thinking too much about my situation and wallowing in self-pity.

I had to accept the nurses I required at night if I was to continue to come home. I wanted to shut the door at night and be with Jill and my children, by myself, like old times, but I had to accept reality. *Step by step, no matter how small. Accept. I'm lucky to be home,* I told myself. Nurses watched me in my room while I slept. It didn't bother me because I had my magic little sleeping pill. I was gone, oblivious to my surroundings.

My private duty nurses were all great, and Patti covered anytime a shift couldn't be filled. But I hated needing someone else, a stranger, in my home, only because it reminded me how disabled I had become. I was dependent on others to defecate, urinate, eat, and breathe. And yet I felt like the same old Shawn. My hope was that my disability would be temporary. These weekends at home made my time at Stan Cassidy more tolerable, but being home didn't make everything perfect — far from it. It reminded me of all the things I missed.

The first morning home, I cried. After the morning wash-up, Jill wheeled me out to the breakfast table. The breakfast nook looks out onto our backyard through bay windows. The woods were active with birds despite the rather foggy day. It would have been a good day to do those chores that needed to be done inside the house or to curl up with a book on the sofa.

The realization that my life had changed hit me hard. *This may not be a transient stage,* I told myself. *This may be it! I may never be able to get out of this chair. I can't even curl up and read a book on the sofa.*

I was overcome with the feeling of being confined to the wheelchair. I felt trapped. It wasn't even that comfortable. My behind was already starting to cry out for relief. I didn't want to go back to bed so soon! *What am I going to do with the rest of the day? I want to move!*

I hung my head and cried; everything seemed so grey. I was thankful my kids weren't up, but as usual, poor Jill became my emotional washcloth. It was hard to express emotion through an eye-gaze board, but I told her that I was just frustrated. Jill cried with me and told me it *wasn't* fair; I didn't deserve this.

I didn't deserve this! That statement reminded me that Pauli didn't deserve her scleroderma; Dorothy didn't deserve her cancer; Susan didn't deserve her multiple sclerosis. It is not a question of who deserves what. I'm not special; things just happen. Many years before, I had read a book by Harold S. Kushner, *When Bad Things Happen to Good People.* It helped me make sense of tragedy involving my patients, and I think his message helped me during these times.

My poor wife had to absorb these emotional outbursts, and we are too close for my emotions not to affect her. I realized this, but I couldn't suppress my feelings in front of her, and the knowledge that I must be causing her sorrow made me feel bad. Any stroke survivor's partner has a heavy load to bear. They have to deal with emotional outbursts and maybe personality changes on top of increased physical demands. The stroke survivor may not act like the same person they married. Usually the marriage is firmly established by the time a stroke occurs, yet more than 50 percent of marriages end in divorce after a stroke.

My emotional outburst quickly passed, and it made me feel better. I spent the rest of the weekend enjoying visits from friends, resting in bed, watching TV, and "talking" to my kids and Jill. Leaving for Fredericton the next day was especially painful. My kids helped me into the car, sliding me along my board. Not a simple task, but once it was accomplished, I left them in the driveway. And as we pulled out, I already missed them. Colin was acting so mature and reliable for a young twenty-year-old man and watching out for his sisters. Beth, such a gentle soul, was in her last year of high school. She might have been having a tough time concentrating on her schoolwork as a result of the sudden change in our family. I felt so sad thinking about my youngest, Tara, in grade eight, waking up tomorrow morning without her mother, eating breakfast by herself, and going to school. I felt so guilty and sad watching my children as they waved goodbye that I burst into tears.

I'm supposed to be the strong one, helping my kids, but they're helping me. They're smiling and waving goodbye, and I'm the one crying. Stop it! Stop it! I wanted to stop crying, but I had no control. I didn't want my children to see me like this. I felt stupid. Jill pulled the car over down the street, out of sight of our home, and wiped my eyes.

My first day back, I quickly became immersed in the daily routine at Stan Cassidy: up shortly after seven, a quick wash-up and tube feed, and then my swallowing exercises at nine with my speech language pathologist. It was good that I was kept busy at Stan Cassidy — less time for thinking. I was still aching to socialize.

Later in the week, as one of the nurses washed me in bed, I heard a story on the radio about a twenty-nine-year-old woman who had died in a motor vehicle accident on the highway. This sad news of a woman I had never met had a huge impact on my mental state for the next few months. Whenever I started to feel sorry for myself, all I had to do was think of this unknown young woman: *I don't deserve to be locked in, but neither did that young woman deserve to die. At least I'm living.*

Another phrase became a mantra around this time: *Shit happens!* Those young men in Vietnam could not have summed it up better to make sense of the mayhem they went through. I would use that phrase to myself, as well as to others when they asked me how I felt about what had happened to me. It just about summed it up for me, too. It prevented me from dwelling on negative thoughts, what-ifs, anger, and self-pity. *Shit happens!*

Sometimes, entertaining things happened with the nursing staff. Kim was a small woman who worked like a hummingbird. It was like she'd taken an overdose of thyroid medication before each shift. She didn't walk; she ran from task to task. I never saw her saunter. She was freakishly strong despite her small stature. She pulled me across my sliding board with minimal effort and easily lifted me up from a lying position to sitting. Larger-statured nurses found this a hard task, especially because of my rigidity, but little Kim flung me around with apparent ease.

One morning it was her turn to suction my tracheotomy and clean it. They were trying not to suction and humidify my trach as often, to see if it would dry up and give me a solid night's sleep. I had spent quite a good night, and for the first time I did get through with no suctioning or humidity. Another nurse had just given me some moist air to loosen the mucus before Kim came in.

I breathed quietly, but as I found out, it was the quiet before the storm. The phlegm had dried out during the night, but there was just as much of it. The trach just didn't sound like it was full.

Kim talked about her dog, her husband, and how nice it was out. She quickly arranged her trach tray, attached the suction tube to the machine, turned the noisy thing on, and dived in.

It worked. She created a cough and quickly removed the suction tube with only a small amount of mucus. "This is curious." Kim said. "You always produce more phlegm than this. You went all night ... perhaps we missed it. I'll go down again."

The first cough had produced little mucus, but now an ominous noise arose from my trach. It sounded like the rumblings of a volcano before it erupts. I heard it and felt it. I was about to spew the mother of all hawkers.

Kim took careful aim, intent on her mission: suction up those goobers or die trying. The sun streamed into my room, making the air close with heat. Kim had her mask on. I imagined it was hot for her, too. I remembered times in the operating room when I was involved in an especially long procedure; each breath seemed hotter than the last as I re-breathed the air that couldn't escape the mask. That first breath outside the operating room felt so good.

I watched as Kim leaned over my trach tube. *Don't do that!* I wanted to yell. Once, a girl had come in to the ER with an apparent drug overdose. We must have been told that she had taken the drugs not too long before admission, because I elected to do a gastric lavage, hoping to get some pills up before they were absorbed. I inserted a large gastric tube down her throat and then poured water into the tube to flush the pills out. I pressed on her stomach, expecting the contents would soon follow. Nothing happened. We turned her on her side and pressed harder. Nothing. I added more water through the tube to her gastric contents and pressed again. Nothing. Pressed harder. Nothing. Remember Elmer Fudd looking down his gun barrel when it didn't fire? Remember what happened to him? I had obviously learned nothing from this cartoon as a youngster. What I hoped to see, I have no idea, but like Elmer, I mindlessly peered down the barrel of the gun — the gastric tube — looking for that mysterious obstruction. Without any provocation, the girl suddenly vomited up her pre-suicide meal. Why would someone contemplating suicide decide to eat ham and eggs before they overdosed? And a good quantity, too!

I stood there with partially digested ham and eggs clinging to my head and clothes while the nurses tried to suppress their laughter. However, I had managed to lavage most of the pills along with the meal, and the patient lived to eat more ham and eggs. My dignity was not so lucky.

I don't want to make light of a serious and far too common presentation to the ER: teen suicide. We successfully saved this girl and arranged for follow-up psychiatric evaluation and care. I hope she found the help she needed and is living a happy, healthy life.

As Kim worked over my trach, I thought of this girl and my mistake. This time the suctioning worked, but it was too copious and thick for a measly suction tube. I coughed out more phlegm than I thought humanly possible in one huge, sudden bark.

Kim held her ground, fine nurse that she is, and took the full disgorgement of my night's rest. Her face, glasses, and hair were plastered with gobs of gross mucus. She bravely continued to work and cleaned off her face only when the necessary tasks were finished.

Kim didn't seem to be aware that her hair also had gobs of phlegm attached to it. I was afraid that, at any minute, an emergency call bell would ring in another patient's room and off she would rush, mindless of her hair looking like she had crawled out of someone's nightmare. I tried to point to her hair, but I couldn't lift my left arm high enough. So I tried to warn her by extending my finger in the direction of the washroom. After another frustrating question-and-blink-the-eyes session, I finally made her understand that she should look at her hair.

Kim was not freaked out when she looked in the mirror. "Oh, that's all right. It happens," she said.

She finished my care calmly and later washed her hair. I noticed that after this, she held her head back whenever she did my trach care. Sensible woman! I think she understood the lesson Elmer Fudd gave us, too!

I was still seeing double because my eye muscles were not working together. My world was fuzzy, compounding my feelings of unreality. Eric, the brainstem stroke survivor who was a year ahead of me in recovery, still had double vision. I started to worry that permanent double vision might also be my fate. Eric and I both wore an eye patch over one eye — using just one eye stopped the double vision — but I found it hot to wear in the summer and wore it infrequently, preferring the diplopia over the heat and sweat.

Each morning upon awakening, I looked at the room number on my door. Instead of seeing a single eight, I saw two of them, telling me nothing had changed. I hoped for so many things each day when I woke up: that I would spontaneously be moving my legs and arms and talking. That I'd surprise the nurses by saying "Good morning!" to them as they entered my room. I imagined they would cover their mouths, astonished, and scream, "Shawn, what …?" Then they'd laugh and we would all cry. I'd thank them all, walk to physio, and repeat the scene with Mereille, Doreen, and Beth, then walk back to my room and pack my bags for home. I knew it would never happen, but I couldn't help dreaming.

One morning, the eights seemed closer together. I looked at the clock. The numbers seemed more defined. Imagination? If improvement had occurred, the rest of the day didn't provide any convincing evidence.

The next day, the eights seemed closer still, and within a matter of a week, my vision was normal. As we drove home the next weekend, I saw the forest clearly. *That's an osprey nest on the electrical tower near Welsford! I thought something was there. The clouds are so clear and distinct in the blue sky!* I smiled all the way home that weekend, although you wouldn't have been able to tell by my expression.

I thought all recovery would be like this and maybe, just maybe, I was on my way. Each week something else would improve. Perhaps next week it would be my left arm, and then the week after, my left leg, and then …

However, no function ever improved as rapidly as my eyes did. The recovery phase of stroke can be cruel. Sometimes improvement can be a tease: you can't duplicate the achievement, or if you can, it finally happens weeks later. Sometimes gains are so painfully slow, and you expend huge amounts of energy for small gains. It is frustrating, heartbreaking work, and you never know if all that effort will bear fruit. But you can't give up! I worked every day and still got improvements in function two years after the stroke. Now, twenty years later, I exercise to maintain function, not expecting any progress, but occasionally I get a surprising new movement.

It was hard to exercise some days. Sometimes there were no improvements for weeks and I felt that there was no point in continuing. Then some function improved — I moved my arm a little farther — and all that work meant something. That was how it went. I often questioned when should I stop trying an exercise that never led to improvements. I guess when those little rewards do stop. When will I know? I don't think anyone can tell me.

I have an obsessive personality, so that helped me to continue even when there were no signs of improvement, but I can easily understand folks who get discouraged and stop trying. I tried to remind myself that I might try and try and still fail but I would certainly fail if I didn't try.

To this day, Jill wants to help when she sees me struggle and it is always tempting to accept her help just to complete whatever task I'm doing. Getting the cap off the toothpaste may seem very insignificant, but it's therapy. If I want to rehabilitate to my full potential, I have to resist getting lazy!

I saw my speech language pathologist, Beth, twice a day. She concentrated on teaching me to swallow again. I could swallow reflexively but not on command, and certainly not well enough to eat or clear saliva. I hated being in bed, but at least when I was flat I didn't drool. When I went out to the lounge, I was aware of saliva flowing from my mouth and down my chin and thought about how I must look. It wasn't just a polite trickle of drool, but an embarrassing, disgusting flood of mouth fluids.

I was very aware then of how disabled I must appear to strangers: an apparently brain-dead, completely paralyzed, drooling man. I imagined them thinking, *Isn't it nice how his family takes him out and talks to him like he's normal?* I felt strangers looking at me, wondering. I wanted to scream at them, *I'm normal! I'm a doctor! I have children! Two months ago, I walked, drove, played guitar, golfed* (badly) *and sang* (again, badly). *I could talk to you about sports, politics, bananas — whatever!* Instead, I could offer them no reaction; I stared and drooled with little expression. If they looked closely, they might have seen my eyes tearing over as I read their minds.

The drooling was so bad it soaked my shirt within half an hour. My chin would get sore and irritated from the saliva. I got so exasperated that I literally put a sock in it. I asked my family to stuff a towel in my mouth to soak up the saliva. If I thought I had looked bad before, now I definitely warranted a second look!

My poor mother stared at me in disbelief when I first asked her to stuff a towel in my mouth. Mom and Dad had just wheeled me out to the lounge to watch TV on the big screen. After a while, tired again of my constant drooling, I asked Mom through the eye-gaze board to put a towel in my mouth. She was not great at using the board, and I could see she thought she had made a mistake. "Ron!" she said to my stepfather. "You see what he's saying. I'm so stupid with this."

Resigning myself to the inevitable, I repeated myself on the board to Dad.

"Well, I think he said, 'Put a towel in my mouth,'" Dad said.

"That's what I thought you said!" Mom exclaimed. "You want me to put a towel in your mouth?"

It occurred to me how strange this request must seem to her, and I began to laugh-cough.

"Why in God's name would someone want a towel shoved in their mouth?" Mom laughed.

Somehow, between coughing fits, I managed to explain my strange request. Mom found a towel, but because she didn't want to hurt me, I ended up with only a corner of the towel in my mouth. I didn't want to confuse things or take the effort to communicate further about my request, so I accepted the small achievement.

One evening, as I sat watching TV with a towel stuffed in my mouth, Pierre, a motor-vehicle-accident victim who had been in a coma for six months, came into the lounge. One side of his body was very damaged, and his better side was not great. His mouth was twisted, and he spoke with a drunk-sounding drawl. His speech was hard to make out, but he said, "Can I watch the weather for a second?"

Gee, the poor guy. Must have had quite a crack-up. Looks bad, I thought. *Must have lost a few marbles from that one!* So thought the man with a towel sticking out of his mouth! A great one to prejudge. Pierre became my friend. His survival and recovery were remarkable, and his tenacity to improve and his outlook on life were inspiring. And best of all, his humour made me choke on more than one occasion. That was the last time I ever prejudged anyone based on first appearance.

I would be only too glad to get rid of the towel. So I approached my sessions with Beth with great interest. She placed cold objects in the back of my mouth, hoping to induce a swallow, but usually nothing happened. Progress was slow.

After weeks of this, I started to produce a weak voluntary swallow. Then I tried to do it on command. Beth would place her hand on my throat and ask me to swallow. I don't even think I can do a swallow on command now! I seemed to have a psychological block, and I became afraid they wouldn't let me eat until I could swallow on command.

It was a great source of frustration for me. I tried to close my eyes and imagine drinking water, but nothing helped. After weeks, Beth asked me to try to swallow twice within a certain time span. It was hard and it took a long time and a lot of practice, but eventually I did it.

Along with these swallowing exercises, Beth also spent time trying to get my facial muscles working. She asked me to frown, smile, pucker, and round my lips. At first, there was no movement — it seemed impossible. But eventually, with time and Beth's persistence, movement occurred. I found this was usually the norm: I experienced no sudden achievement and thus no positive reinforcement. There was no day when I screamed, "I can move it!" The return of movement was so gradual that I could not perceive it. When did I first move my lips? Hard to pinpoint. It happened, but when?

It would have been nice to have a few eureka moments. Most of my goals were achieved without any fanfare. One day, two years after my stroke, I turned off a light in the bathroom. Before that, I couldn't raise my arm high enough to reach the switch, so I had used an extension attached to it. When did I start raising my arm that high? I have no idea.

Beth tried to induce my facial muscles to work by placing ice over the muscle she wanted to move. Eventually my mouth opened a crack and I was amazed to find my tongue did not work. The things we take for granted! I could not get my tongue out of my mouth.

Over at occupational therapy, we were having problems finding a suitable wheelchair seat. In all the seats we tried, I lasted only a few hours before my bottom cried in pain.

Doreen also kept changing the controls on the power chair to challenge my left hand. She stretched my hands and exercised them, and after weeks of trying, my left hand started to move. We spent time working on making a fist, releasing the grip, and trying to pinch with the index finger and thumb. I could see small weekly improvements thanks to repetition, persistence, and patience. But no eureka.

One day, Doreen had me pick up little plastic mice from one container with my left hand and place them in another. It was a Thursday morning; I remembered that on Thursday mornings before my stroke, I often did minor surgery. In fact, the day of my whiplash, I had removed a basal cell carcinoma from a man's face. Now my left hand refused to co-operate. If I managed to raise my hand high enough to grasp the mice, it took all my strength to move my arm over and let go. In my frustration, I thought of how easy it had been to remove that basal cell just two months before. Now I couldn't move stupid plastic mice.

Those mice depressed me. I hated their stupid tails, bright colours, and plastic smell. I begrudged the sunny summer day while I sat in this therapy room trying — and usually failing — to pick up plastic mice.

I later realized how important those mice were; I didn't really hate them. But it was hard. It was hard to not feel sorry for myself when I wanted to be golfing, swimming, boating, working, anything on that nice day. I did not want to feel sorry for myself again. *It's just tough luck! Remember, shit happens!* I told myself. *More people than you are not able to enjoy summer days.*

In physiotherapy, Mereille concentrated on my sitting balance and posture. One of the first things she did was to strap me to a tilt table that could be gradually shifted to an upright position. People can get quite dizzy when first using it, but thankfully, I never had this problem. As I got closer to ninety degrees, the feeling of falling forward increased. I knew I was perfectly safe, but that didn't stop the terror. My sense of balance was terribly damaged from the stroke.

The tilt table also allowed me to experience weight on my feet, and I started to move my left arm and hand toward my face on this device. At first, I could move my arm only to my waist, then to my belly, then weeks later, to my chest. My right arm showed no inclination to move.

It was on the tilt table that my legs first showed signs of movement. Mereille had me bend my knees and then, using my thigh muscles, come back up again. It was a struggle. My thighs burned. Mereille asked me to go lower. *I can't do it*, I thought. But down I went, to the verge of collapse, and back up I struggled. Physiotherapy is hard work. Nothing comes easy, and failure is common. I wanted to improve so badly; I welcomed this scheduled torture for as long as they could take me.

Actually, that's a lie: I never found physiotherapy a torture. It was hard, yes, but never torturous. Mereille was always cheerful and encouraging. I became dependent on her and demonstrated this one day.

I was about to lose Mereille for three weeks while she went on vacation. Of course, I knew everyone took vacation, and naturally, I would be sad to see her go. But in my emotionally labile state, I cried. Horrors! Right in the gym, in front of everyone, Dr. Jennings had decided to bawl his eyes out. I knew everyone here was used to people with stroke and their emotional fragility, but this was me! I knew Mereille understood, but I felt humiliated. Nothing made me feel more abnormal than crying. I quickly left the gym, and no sooner was I out the door than the crying stopped.

The physiatrist, the doctor who specialized in rehabilitation, usually visited me in the mornings before my therapies started. He was a tall fellow with an average build, dark curly hair, and a moustache. He always took the time to understand me. He knew how to use the eye-gaze board well, so I could talk to him. At first, he seemed very serious — probably because I seemed so serious. It was hard to joke and reveal my true personality using the eye-gaze board. Later, when I could talk, I found him very friendly and approachable about any of my concerns.

At that time, my main concern was getting the trach out and removing the tube from my stomach. *When? When?* I asked. Of course, it was hard for him to say, or perhaps he didn't want me to hear the truth. I thought in terms of weeks, but he probably knew it would be months.

He was well aware of how I was doing; I think he relied on reports from Mereille and Doreen at the weekly case conference, where they discussed every patient. They ran a very good inter-professional health-team approach at Stan Cassidy. He always knew how I was progressing, but up to this point, he had seemed evasive in answering my questions.

One morning in July, he was very frank. He told me I probably wouldn't learn to walk. I looked at him and nodded. I probably looked like I was taking this news very calmly, aided by my expressionless face, but inside my stomach knotted, my heart missed a beat, and my emotions froze. My somewhat good mood tumbled down as I looked reality in the face again.

I didn't like what I saw when I considered the possibilities for the future. I didn't believe I could live in a wheelchair forever — it was too uncomfortable, too confining. *He doesn't know me*, I thought. *I've always fought back. I've been able to achieve anything if I put my mind to it. I've never failed. What he is saying is probably true of most people in my position. They probably wouldn't learn to walk, but I will!*

The physiatrist later told me that based upon my progress up to that point, he thought walking was an unlikely achievement. I am thankful he was always honest with me, but at that time, I convinced myself he had given me the worst-case scenario. *He probably doesn't want me getting false hopes*, I reasoned. *I'm a physician; I know how we work.*

The sinking feeling didn't last too long. I thought I'd improve at a quicker pace once the trach was removed. I requested and obtained scientific studies on brainstem strokes from my physiatrist. The news wasn't good. From these readings, I discovered that most brainstem stroke victims died. Of those who did survive, the majority lived with a fair degree of disability. A small number regained normal function. I noticed that the average age of brainstem stroke patients tended to be younger than that for cerebral stroke, which was by far the more common type.

The hope of complete recovery dwindled. Yet I thought, *Maybe I'll be somewhere in between. At least I'll walk.*

Nurses still had to do everything for me. Having another person wipe my eyes was difficult; they usually wiped too softly. It is hard for anyone to gauge how hard or softly to wipe someone else's eye. Later in the day, the sleep from my eyes would fall back in or dissolve, giving me an intense burning sensation.

Another difficulty was where to place the call bell. At least now I could use one. It was a large button that had to be pressed. Usually they pinned it to my pillow and I had to turn my head to activate it. The problem was, because the head of my bed was elevated to help me breathe, I sometimes slid down during the night, and the bell ended up above my head, leaving me no way to call a nurse. I spent many hours uncomfortable, wanting to turn, or wet because my condom catheter had slipped off.

One night was particularly uncomfortable. I woke up with vomit in my mouth. I felt ill and retched again, but not all the vomit came up; some stayed in my throat. I was having a hard time trying to bring it up or swallow it, and it was burning. This was the one night they had deflated the trach, taking the air out of the bulb that holds the trach in place in my windpipe, so I was scared I might aspirate the vomit.

When I tried to call the nurse, I found the call bell was now above my head. I tried wiggling my head to bring the bell down, but the pillow wouldn't budge. I couldn't make any sound with my arms or legs, so I blew out of my trach as hard as I could, hoping to create a noise, but my attempts were feeble owing to my small lung capacity. I couldn't cough on demand; I tried but nothing came.

I continued to be nauseated and thought I might vomit at any time, heightening my fear of aspiration. The burning in my throat and mouth continued. I was alone, with no roommate.

It was the only time I was ever frightened at the centre. I spent a good hour in this state, lying in my own vomit, trying to swallow, afraid I might vomit again, and trying to make a sound. Finally, a nurse came in on her regular rounds.

Later, I became able to move my left hand enough to press the bell. Later still, I had enough strength in my left thumb to use a regular call bell if it was pinned nearby. My predicament that night never happened again, but those first two months were difficult. I hope a better system to allow locked-in patients to call for help is available now or will be devised in the future.

Gradually, I developed a condition that became my main obstacle to rehabilitation, my main source of pain, my heartbreak: rigidity. It started so slowly, I barely noticed.

When a severe injury occurs to the spinal cord, no messages get to the muscles. The lower motor neurons — the nerve cells in the spinal cord that connect directly to specific muscles — tell the muscles to turn on. For an unknown reason, some muscles are turned on more than others; as a result, the arms tend to be flexed (bent at the elbow and held into the body) and the legs extended (straight and held together).

Betty, a physiotherapy assistant at Stan Cassidy who became my friend, stretched my arms and legs every morning before physio. Some movements were painful, some were not so bad, but all were very necessary, and it became as routine as brushing my teeth. At first this occurred in my room after breakfast. Later, it was in the gym, just before my physiotherapy. I grew fond of Betty; we communicated somehow, and I learned about her family and she mine. The best word to describe Betty would be *gentle*. It is hard to stretch someone to the point of pain and still be described as gentle, but that was Betty. I wish I could have talked to her better, but we did all right.

When we started to do the stretches in the gym, Esmond, another staff member, joined us. The exercises took quite a lot of time, so to shorten the activity, we started to perform the stretching with two people at the same time. Esmond was a middle-aged, well-built fellow with white hair who was always smiling. He worked as an assistant in physiotherapy, occupational therapy, and recreation. He amused me with his tales of horses, home, cars, and past experiences. He always had a cheerful story to tell. Esmond would take one leg and Betty the other, and off they would go. We called it synchronized physiotherapy!

As July ended, I had not progressed as far as I had expected. I still had hope that my rehabilitation success would accelerate once the trach and feeding tube were removed. When I moved, the trach made me cough, and my abdomen was sore from the feeding tube rubbing against the edge of the opening. *Maybe soon they'll be gone*, I thought.

CHAPTER 16
AUGUST

In August, the hot weather persisted, and I was still quite the fashion model in my white stockings and shorts. I continued to breathe through the tracheotomy tube in my neck and was nourished via the stomach tube.

The hot weather teased me into thinking about drinking water. The glass of water I imagined was poured over ice cubes from a large glass pitcher with moisture beads clinging to the outside and slices of lemon floating on top. The image made my throat quiver in anticipation.

After I was done tormenting myself with this vision, the thing I most wanted was a cola drink. I don't know why; I'm not a big cola drinker, but I desperately wanted a taste of that dark pop. I suppose it was the wetness, coldness, fizz, and taste — all of those sensations at once. I missed the sense of taste and the act of chewing.

My dietitian, Sharon, knowing that I wanted that taste, made cola ice cubes and allowed me a small amount. They didn't trust me with ice cubes on my own. This was one reason I liked speech therapy sessions, because Beth often used ice cubes to help me swallow. It felt so good in my mouth!

Besides thirst, bugs were another torment during the summer. If a fly happened to enter my room, I could count on a few moments of fun. I was convinced that if there was only one fly in the whole building, it would find me when my tube feeding started.

A fly would land on my face (usually my nose, as it's quite prominent!) and take a little walkabout. This was most annoying, so I tried shaking my head, which I could do slowly by this time, to get it off. This bothered the timid ones, but it had no effect on most. They liked to saunter about and then take a curious look in my nostrils, calculating the risk versus reward of entering. Thankfully, they were basically cowards and not one ventured in.

Around this time, I had a dream that a fly went down my trach and into my throat and laid eggs, and later, out came a writhing mass of maggots! I guess my unwanted little guests *were* affecting me. They landed on my feeding tube, looking for a way in. They crawled along my bare arms, tickling me. Unable to swat them, I was a big playground for flies. Jill bought two fly swatters and kept guard. The nurses became expert marksmen on my behalf.

It might sound like the centre was dirty, but that was far from the truth. The flies got in because of the two large sets of automatic doors at the entrance, which were always opening and closing. There were not many flies; they all just seemed to like me and told their friends, "Hey, there's a guy in there who doesn't mind us taking a walkabout. C'mon!"

Flies were harmless, but the blackflies and mosquitoes were not. Outside, I was fair game. A mosquito would land on my arm and I would helplessly watch as it chose its site, then filled its belly with my blood. Word soon got around among them, too. Jill would catch me flashing my eyes for help, but it was often too late.

Worse than the mosquitoes were the blackflies, which came around in June. Those suckers hurt! And worse again were the horseflies. They elicited a most vigorous shake of my head and a *whoosh* sound from my trach, my "Mayday, mayday!" call.

Then there were the creepy-crawlies, harmless for the most part but bent on making my nightmares real. A spider once crawled up my white stockings and disappeared under my shorts, never to be seen again. I assumed that after it had had a bit of fun at my expense, it left. Often, some creepy varmint would take a shortcut up my wheelchair and onto my arm. If an insect landed on the back of my neck, it was bad; I couldn't see what it was and didn't know if it had crawled under my shirt or flown away. I didn't like what I could not see.

I felt helpless. Any insect that chose to explore my body had free rein until seen by Jill. I had never been afraid of insects when I was able-bodied and had the option of picking them off. I was not so brave now that I was an insect amusement park.

August was my month of impatience. The routine of hospital life, my slow progress, my inability to eat, and my trach all frustrated me. My trach did not behave. The doctor had ordered the nurses to deflate the cuff that surrounded the tube and held it in place in my trachea. They did this to make sure I was not aspirating mucus from my throat, yet it caused another problem: every time I moved, the tube moved in my airway and I coughed. I felt that my coughing was slowing my progress; each time I tried to turn or bend, I was struck with a coughing spasm and had to stop that activity.

My trachea seemed to be more sensitive than those of most people around me or in my experience. The doctor was waiting for my trachea to settle down and produce less mucus as a sign that it was okay to remove the tube. It never did. I continued to produce a lot of mucus until the day they took it out.

I also had to demonstrate that I could breathe with the trach corked or covered. The first time I tried, I lasted a breath or two before I sent the cap flying across the room. I failed each time, and when the head nurse, Louise, indicated that was enough for the day, I would be mad at myself. I had thought I could do it. Another failure! I wanted the trach removed so badly. I thought that once it was gone, presto, I would start talking and eating and maybe even improve physically. I hoped the removal of my trach would be the key to instant improvement. If only stroke rehabilitation were so easy. I knew the truth, but I chose to hope for an easier way out.

I was sure I could talk without the trach. The words were right there in my head, and Sandy, a friend who was a neurologist, had said my speech centre had been spared. The first time that Louise capped my trach and asked me to speak, I was shocked. In my head I said, "How are you?," but out came a feeble "Aaah."

No matter, I thought. *I'm just out of practice.* I did believe this, but the doctor part of me said, *See, I told you so! Why do you keep thinking you're different from any patient you've ever seen?* I guess it was because, although I had seen plenty of strokes, I had never had a patient with a brainstem stroke — maybe they were different. Besides, I had no experience as a patient. But the reality was that I was a patient now. I thought like a patient. I *did* leave my black bag in my truck; it found its way to me only on occasion.

I tried to believe the reason for my lack of air support and my inability to breathe around the tube when it was corked was that my trachea was too narrow. The real reason was that my vital capacity, or the amount of air that I used to breathe, had been greatly reduced. My breathing muscles were very weak. I would have to be patient, to practise, and to believe that someday

I would be able to breathe with my trach capped. But it was so impossible at first that I couldn't imagine ever being able to do so. I was frustrated.

Gradually, I tolerated the trach being capped for longer periods of time. It took more than a month, but eventually I was breathing through my nose. One of my most happy days took place in September when they removed my tracheotomy tube, because I never grew used to it or to the constant suctioning.

I also grew impatient with the feeding tube. My skin was inflamed where it entered my abdomen. I wanted to start eating, and I grew tired of my inability to swallow.

For two or three weeks toward the end of August, I became nauseated with every tube feed. I felt very ill. The nausea would begin about an hour after the tube feed had started. I often implored the nurses to stop the feeds early or skip them altogether. One day, I asked for and received only clear fluids. I'm sure I drove Sharon, my dietitian, crazy. We all know that doctors make lousy patients.

I felt like I was being force fed, trapped in an involuntary, nasty situation. I knew I needed the nutrition and that I had no option, but I couldn't take it anymore. As soon as the milky concoction started flowing through the tube, I knew what would soon follow: bloating, cramps, nausea, sweaty palms and forehead, and nervousness.

I thought it might be dumping syndrome, a condition whereby the stomach empties too fast into the intestine without fully digesting the food. I had no medical reason for this condition, and although it's talked about a lot, it's quite rare. Perhaps I had an ulcer or reflux? There was no pain, but I did regurgitate occasionally and it did taste terrible. Reflux was possible, but I thought the nausea was worse than would be expected for reflux disease. Perhaps my symptoms were psychological. Perhaps just the appearance of the creamy, milk-like substance was triggering a learned food aversion and making me ill. The nurses tried covering the tube feed with a bag but that didn't help. Travis, a student working in recreation, pasted pictures of beautiful young women over the tube feed. That didn't work, although it might have helped my mood!

I wondered if I was depressed; certainly, the cyclic nausea made me feel down. A depressed mood is different from a clinical depression, but which one was it? *I have reason to be depressed*, I thought. *My world has been turned upside down.* Depression is common after strokes. I couldn't be happy about my situation. I had other symptoms, too, including lack of interest and fatigue.

I decided later that depression wasn't the problem. I slept fairly well, although with the help of pills, and between the bouts of nausea, I felt quite well.

I finally decided it was probably irritable bowel syndrome (IBS), a very common condition. I've seen many people with it, and I was prone to experiencing symptoms of IBS under stress. It's not dangerous, and there is nothing abnormal in the diagnostic tests, but I found it more disabling than one might think. I have been nauseated from food or the flu, but IBS made me feel worse than that. I have never felt more ill than when my IBS acted up.

IBS is definitely worse when one is anxious, leading many to believe it is a psychological disease manifested by slow or irregular activity of the bowel. When one is relaxed, the bowels actually work harder; when one is upset, bowel activity is weak and sluggish, which leads to bloating, cramps, irregularity, and nausea. It's a difficult condition to treat because it's really only a variation of normal physiology. There are many different remedies, none of them hugely successful, which usually means there is no cure. My physiatrist was on vacation, so I told his replacement my suspicion and asked him to prescribe a small dose of anticholinergic. This had worked for me in the past, although it hadn't been that satisfactory for many of my patients. What works for some does not work for everyone with this disease.

I felt better within a day. I don't know if it was the medication that helped or time. Maybe I'd just had a prolonged intestinal virus, because I did have some diarrhea during this period. I couldn't stop trying to diagnose my own condition and just leave it with my physicians. I suppose that's probably true for most doctors who become patients. It's hard to turn off the symptom-and-diagnosis mode of thinking and become neutral and dependent on another doctor's opinion. I hope I didn't give my treating physicians too much grief; I don't think I did.

My ability to urinate without a catheter improved. I could tell now when I needed to urinate, but not until it was urgent. When I needed to go, I needed to go! There had better be a nurse handy, ready to whip down my shorts and diaper and put the urinal in place. It wasn't critical if I couldn't hold the urge, because I had a diaper on, but I was trying hard to train my bladder.

I found urinating while sitting down difficult. Often the nurse didn't pull the diaper down far enough — I assume because she was afraid of crushing some other things of mine — and the urinal would be pointing skyward. Physics dictates that this won't work; I would have thought she'd known that! Alas, unable to verbalize my concern or hold my urine any longer, I challenged physics, only to lose every time.

As time passed, I gained better control and discarded the diapers. I wasn't confident in my bladder control until the following spring. Until then, I needed the occasional change of pants and suffered the occasional wounded ego, once again illustrating that nothing improves quickly in stroke recovery.

I was frustrated also by my inability to look after my own personal hygiene. I was dependent on the nurses for everything: washing, drying, shaving, brushing my teeth, everything, down to washing my genitalia and wiping my behind. I was incapable of attempting any of these tasks, so I couldn't play the grumpy patient and say, "Here, let me do that!" I had no resources to allow me to act independent, insolent, or difficult.

Nevertheless, I did become difficult in one area: the washing of my hair. It seems so petty when I look back on it, but at that time, it was important to me. My hair is blond and thin and tends to get oily within a day. I wanted my hair washed every morning before I got up. They do this by using a shampoo tray in bed, a clumsy procedure that is quite time consuming. The nurses were very busy in the morning, trying to get everyone ready for breakfast at eight, so they often didn't have time to do anything extra. Usually, they did give me a shampoo, probably disrupting their schedule, but if they couldn't, I silently sulked.

It didn't really matter if my hair got washed or not — who was I seeing? What did it matter if my hair was a little greasy for a day? I had to admit, I had no logical reason for this compulsion, but for more than twenty years it had been my habit to have a shower as soon as I awoke. I think the desire to have my hair washed was an attempt to hold on to something I missed, some normalcy in my life. Everything had changed; nothing was familiar — urinating, having a bowel movement, brushing my teeth, combing my hair, eating, talking — nothing. But really, having my hair washed was such an insignificant action in the complete picture of my life change that I'm surprised it bothered me so much at the time.

I was able to let go of this obsession and, subsequently, my inner anger and resentment, after I'd engaged in the above self-analysis. I have found in my life that honest self-reflection helps me to deal with inner turmoil. I sometimes need to step back and think about why I'm feeling the way I am about a certain situation. The trick is to remember to self-reflect after the anger, anxiety, sadness, or whatever negative emotion is experienced.

The nursing staff must have thought I was vain — and maybe I am. One nurse in particular would have understood if it was vanity. Louise had warned me about her the first day I came to Stan Cassidy. She told me there would be a nurse who would make the sign of the cross on my chest when she applied underarm antiperspirant. I had never heard of this religious custom and didn't know what to expect.

Linda, a francophone, was the nurse who had this strange habit. I grew fond of Linda over the months. She was very particular as to how her patients were cleaned up and dressed for the day — apparently my colour coordination was non-existent. When I progressed to being able to shave myself, my initial attempts were poor. Linda couldn't stand to let me go around like that, so she finished the job. It didn't bother me that I wasn't perfectly shaven, but if the results didn't meet Linda's standards, even when I thought they were finally acceptable, she shaved more. There was no hair on my face but plenty of razor burn!

Linda's fussiness amused me and her nursing skills impressed me. I asked her how she came to be called Linda, a very English name, I thought, for a French girl to be given. Apparently, at the time of her birth in the northern part of New Brunswick, it was a common name for French girls. Her smile and spirit helped me through some troubled times.

Not far behind my frustrations were worries. Although I had hope that my condition would improve, I realized there was a real possibility of staying severely handicapped. The probability of not being able to practise medicine loomed as a real threat.

A new doctor in the area wanted to buy my medical supplies and equipment, but selling implied I would not be returning to practise. It was hard for me to finally agree to sell. I had spent more than twenty years with a stethoscope around my neck or in my pocket, and this instrument was such a part of me that I sometimes found, to my embarrassment, that I had a stethoscope around my neck in a store. It felt strange not to be wearing a stethoscope and difficult to accept that I might never use one again.

I was not worried about my office expenses because I had insurance that paid the rent, ongoing office expenses, and the salary of Leah, my receptionist. My personal disability insurance had started that month. But doubts nagged me. Would it be enough money to meet all my expenses? Had I considered that I had one child in college and another soon to go? What would Leah do now if I couldn't return to work? I worried about the costs of renovating my home to make it wheelchair accessible.

I didn't vocalize (funny term, since I was mute!) my financial worries to Jill; she had enough problems. I knew it was better to share my concerns with someone, but I kept them to myself.

I would have welcomed a chance to talk with someone about my finances. The interprofessional team at Stan Cassidy included a social worker, and I had witnessed them privately talking to other patients, yet they had never approached me. Did the social worker assume that because I was a doctor, I had no financial worries or needs? It was true that I was in a much better financial position than most of my fellow patients, but I bet my worries were just as troublesome even if they were different in scale. I know the social worker would have readily interacted with me if I had asked, and my accountant at home would have visited, so it is my fault, really. I could have easily eased my anxiety by reaching out.

Despite being sick, frustrated, and worried, I remained hopeful. I was hopeful because I showed weekly signs of improvement. I felt life returning to my left arm. Each week I could move my fingers better, my hand closer to my face or away from my body, in every parameter. My legs were holding me up better. I was reaching my goals nearly every week, so I was optimistic.

Despite this optimism, I never strayed too far from reality. I had to face undeniable truths: my physiatrist's opinion that I would never walk and the lack of significant improvement after three months, including in my speech and eating. My brother, Duane, kept saying my right hand was just a few weeks behind my left. I listened in frustration to his attempt to keep me positive, thinking, *You do realize, Duane, I've been here almost three months now.* No, I never lost sight of reality from June or July on, but I had hope.

In stroke recovery, the greatest improvement occurs within three months, and although I wasn't improving at the rate I had expected, I had reason to hope. I read and people told me that brainstem strokes were different from cerebral strokes; the improvement tended to happen over a longer time frame. I hoped my information was correct, because I had no experience with a brainstem stroke. I chose to think positively and I had no reason to believe my improvement would stop now.

Frustrations are inherent in all occupations, and indeed in all facets of life. We learn to cope. As society demands more from us, as the speed of interactions increases, so do our stress levels. We have to remember that no one is getting off easy. Nurses, teachers, lawyers, housewives, doctors, car mechanics, store owners, farmers — no one gets a break. I always tried to remember the old saying about walking a mile in someone else's shoes. I think we need to realize that we all have frustrations and stress — different types, different degrees, but we all have trials in our day-to-day lives.

As a doctor, one of my ongoing frustrations involved the business aspect of running a practice. I had trained to be a doctor, yet I also became a small-business owner by owning a practice. I tried to be interested in payrolls, deductions, expenditures, benefits, and balance sheets, but I usually passed these tasks off to Jill.

I was lucky: she actually did them. I called her my office manager/ nurse, paid her a salary, and dodged a major frustration. God bless her; she didn't like these jobs any better than I did.

The politics of medicine, in-hospital territory wars, government-doctor relationships — these all frustrated me. I wasn't good at speaking or leading, but I didn't have to be; there were other doctors much more dynamic than I who eventually said what I thought. I was a soldier. I would sit on any committee, investigate, or do a study, but not lead.

I found it difficult and frustrating trying to keep abreast of the ever-changing practice of medicine. I loved the study of medicine, keeping current, and reading about new studies, but it was hard with a busy practice. The economics of running a practice got so demanding that taking time off for education became difficult.

The actual practice of medicine — the only thing I wanted to do — was smooth. However, the majority of diseases were life-style induced, and I admit that at first, I would be frustrated when patients did not heed my advice. Eventually, I chose not to allow the bad lifestyle habits of my patients bother me. I gave them the facts, and if they chose to ignore them, that was their business. I always lectured those at risk about lack of exercise, smoking, the dangers of eating a high-fat diet, and the benefits of including more fibre or fruits and vegetables in their diet. I tried to keep up my attack but with the attitude of not becoming frustrated when my advice fell on deaf ears. It was their choice. I did my job, and a few patients did benefit from my advice; that was reward enough.

Now, my frustration with my slow rate of improvement was reinforced by my knowledge that the window of time for the greatest progress after a stroke was rapidly closing. I had learned in life and in my medical practice that we can't let irritations eat us up. We have to do our best and just accept that sometimes the effort won't be enough to affect the outcome.

CHAPTER 17
CANCER

Cancer did frustrate me. As the saying goes, it can be beaten if detected early. I took it as a challenge to try to detect cancer early and as a defeat when a patient died of cancer. Cancers of the pancreas and ovary are particularly hard to discover early because these organs are deep inside the body and the cancer can spread without any warning symptoms.

Barbara was an elegant, pretty lady in her fifties who worked as a legal secretary. She was single, I suspect because she was so devoted to the care of her mother, who had severe asthma. Her mother required frequent hospitalizations, aerosols at home, and constant reassurance. This was before the advancements in asthma care we have today. Despite her asthma, Barbara's mother lived to a ripe old age before succumbing to heart failure.

A few years after her mother died, Barb married a fine fellow who had recently lost his wife to cancer. Their home was located on the edge of the Kennebecasis River, with a sandy beach in front. I couldn't imagine a more idyllic setting, and she deserved it after devoting her life to the care of her mother.

One morning, not long after their wedding, she came in to see me, complaining of vague lower-abdominal cramps. I did a pelvic exam as part of my investigation to find the possible cause. I felt my stomach knot up as I palpated her pelvic area. Instead of empty space and a compliant vaginal wall, all I could feel was hard, fibrous tissue. The rectal exam revealed the same result. I felt sick as I clicked into my professional mode and reeled off the tests and consults I would be ordering. I knew this was not good, and it wasn't: she had widespread metastatic cancer of the ovary. Within a few months, I was managing her palliative care at home in that idyllic setting on the river. Her husband looked after her carefully at home with the love and devotion she deserved until she died.

Each time I drove up to their home to look in on Barb, the beautiful surroundings saddened me. She, more than anyone I had ever known, deserved to be walking on that beach instead of dying, because she had sacrificed her own happiness to care for her mother. Barb would have appreciated that big old tree, the waves, the fall sky, the colours, the smells. Where was the fairness? I think it was this death that prompted me to read Harold Kushner's book *When Bad Things Happen to Good People*.

Even when you think you've done everything right, cancer can rise out of nowhere and bite. Sarah was in her sixties. Her husband had died a few years before of emphysema, but she had managed to put her grief behind her and was quite active. I remember her always having a smile and being eager to laugh.

I performed a breast exam and found nothing alarming. She was due for a routine mammogram, which was performed and reported as negative. These investigations were completed in the spring, and I expected to not see her until the following spring. However, she returned in September with a red lump on her breast. At first glance, I thought perhaps it was an abscess, but it felt solid when I touched it. Cancer? No! We had checked her just a few months before. But if it was cancer, it must have been in an early stage.

The lump did prove to be cancerous and despite surgery, chemotherapy, and radiation, it got away from us. Sarah died about a year later. I tried to relive my examination that preceded the cancer. *I know I was careful! I didn't feel anything suspicious, but it must have been there. Or was it?* I felt frustrated; I had done everything right and still cancer had beaten us! I used this story often in the following years to illustrate to women that they should not depend upon my yearly breast exam and the mammogram. It is so important that women conduct their own monthly breast exams, because they will often detect a troublesome area before a doctor will. Cancer can be very aggressive.

I have many more stories about cancer victims, but you get the point. Other diseases frustrated me, too, but not as much as cancer.

I had gotten used to frustrations in life. I tried to react not with anger but with acceptance. The trach, the tube feedings, my lack of progress, and other matters might have been frustrating, but I accepted and tolerated them and swore that I would improve.

CHAPTER 18
LATE AUGUST

I turned forty-six on August 27, and some positive things started to happen by then. One morning, Beth and Doreen took me to the Dr. Everett Chalmers Regional Hospital, the main hospital in Fredericton, for swallowing tests, where doctors would watch me swallow via X-ray video. My performance pleased them, but they seemed to indicate that there was room for improvement. I was disappointed when they stopped the tests; I thought it meant more months of tube feed, but I was wrong. Later that week, I had my first meal.

I was excited. It was lunchtime and Jill, Doreen, and Beth took me to the occupational therapy kitchen for my meal. This was the last time I ate alone, because all patients who could were expected to eat together in the main cafeteria. This was part of the therapy to introduce newly disabled people to normal social situations. But I was thankful to be eating alone because I was anxious. Would I be able to swallow? I envisioned choking and food flying across the room.

I surprised myself by holding the spoon quite normally on my first attempt to do so left handed. However, I struggled to lift my hand up to my mouth while trying to keep the spoon level. I tried different angles and positions until finally the spoon reached my mouth. A bib was placed around my neck and I was ready. Anxiety started to build. My stomach didn't feel hungry, but I hadn't experienced a hunger pain in more than three months, so I wasn't concerned. I felt like an athlete in the blocks awaiting the start of a race; I had trained so hard and for so long just for this moment. I was determined to succeed, but I was ready for failure.

All negative thoughts evaporated from my mind as Sharon brought in my lunch: chicken and rice soup, blended with bread crumbs so that it had a very thick consistency. The smell! I could actually smell *real* food. My taste buds had been deprived for three months and I *would not* fail. They adjusted my elbow so it rested on a table, making it easier for my spoon to reach my mouth.

I'm surprised I didn't cry with the first spoonful. The taste — chicken, salt, pepper — burst in my mouth. I'm not exaggerating; the taste actually *burst*! I had never tasted anything as glorious as that chicken and rice soup. It may not have looked appetizing, but I was ready to defend it like a dog with a bone if anyone tried to take it from me. I managed to swallow without choking and my stomach gladly accepted its first real food in more than three months. Beth, Doreen, Sharon, and Jill watched me closely as I happily ate as much as they dared give me.

Learning to eat again was not easy — it was downright frustrating at times — but I was so thankful to be weaning off of tube feeds that I never became discouraged.

Micheline, the recreation director, was anxious for me to attend an outing. Stan Cassidy Centre has a bus for wheelchairs, and twice a week patients are encouraged to go out with the group to a mall, movie, restaurant, or some other activity. A break in the daily routine at the centre was a treat, but the outings also had an important therapeutic function: integrating newly disabled people back into society.

Before my trach was removed, I was aware of this fact and eager to go with my fellow patients, but at the same time I was anxious about harming someone with my missile-prone trach cap. When I coughed or laughed, the trach cap flew in any random direction, and I was honestly afraid of hitting someone in the mall. I was sure people would be quite grossed out and upset if this happened to them. The possibility seemed real enough that I had chosen not to attempt any trips yet.

Now that my trach had been removed, I did not hesitate to go out with the group. Some newly disabled people are afraid to be seen in public at first, but not me. I was curious to experience the reactions: Would people stare? Look out of the corner of their eye? Would they be afraid to speak to us?

My first outing was to a mall. I was excited about getting out for an evening; for the last three months, I had been only in hospitals or at home. Esmond, the recreational assistant, loaded us onto the bus for our journey. The others made comments about the weather, what they were going to do at the mall, who was going with whom. I listened. I shared their enthusiasm but could not demonstrate it. I again felt locked out, observing but not actively involved.

I was not anxious as we embarked on my debut into society. Instead, I was joyous, a step closer to normalcy. I felt a comradeship with this group of disabled people. Some were in power chairs, a few in manual chairs, some walked, and some were just bewildered. A few were old, a few were young, but we shared common experiences and that gave us our bond.

As we entered the mall, a thought occurred to me: I entered it not only as a doctor, husband, and father, but also, for the first time, as a disabled person. I was still the doctor, husband, and father, but I had a new identity and the new label overshadowed all the others. Now, first and foremost, I was a disabled person. It was not how I saw myself but how others saw me. I knew I was disabled — the denial phase was long over — but that night, among all those able-bodied people, I *felt* disabled.

I had not experienced this type of activity in a while, so many people scurrying to the next shop, talking, laughing, or looking straight ahead, intent upon their goal, doing what mall people do. But they were not looking at me! No one glanced my way. I was not as unique as I thought.

Instead of the mall people looking at me, it was I who looked at them. I was fascinated, watching so many people walk with such ease. I studied how they were doing it: *Flex the hips, raise the knee — it doesn't have to be very high. So effortless! Why can't I learn to do that? Attention, all Kmart shoppers; attention, all Kmart shoppers: get down on your knees and be thankful that you can walk! Do they realize how wonderful it is to be able to walk?*

Of course they didn't. Had I ever been thankful for the gift of walking? No, I hadn't thought about it. And I realized I had been like the mall people: I never saw people in wheelchairs. I think we are so conditioned not to stare at anyone who is different from us that we soon don't see the wheelchairs. Now that I am in a wheelchair, I'm aware of other people in wheelchairs. There are a lot of us out there! I obviously did not see them when I was able-bodied.

Children are curious and innocent, and children in the mall did look at me. I welcomed their attention. However, most were already indoctrinated by their parents not to stare, and they watched me from the corner of their eye. I wanted to talk to them. I always sang and played with the little folks in my office to ease their anxiety about going to the doctor. At first, my antics with my little patients might have been contrived, but soon it became natural. Acting like a child is a delight — everyone should do it daily. The children of my practice gave me joy; I hope in some small way I repaid them.

So I was used to children and wanted to interact with them. But they hid behind their mothers' skirts, afraid of this creature that stared at them with no expression on his face (by this time I could manage a faint smile, but it was fleeting and pretty pathetic). He had a hole in his neck and hardly moved. Perhaps this was the bogeyman!

I knew how I looked in their eyes, so, sadly, I tried to ignore them. But they amazed me more than their parents did: they spun, they skipped, they jumped and, still in midair, twirled about and landed on their feet facing the opposite way. Amazing! Little movements that I had never thought about or had once taken for granted now fascinated me. The body's ability to synchronize balance and the whole assortment of minute movements that must occur in order to jump and twirl in one motion became incredible to me. It's true that we never appreciate what we've got until it's gone.

So it was I who stared at the mall people. They basically ignored me, exactly the opposite of what I had been expecting. I have never encountered rudeness or insensitivity from the able-bodied population. I had read about it and was ready, but it has rarely happened. I have received only polite gestures, sometimes to a fault. I have never been ignored by a sales clerk or spoken about like I wasn't there. I have been spoken down to, as if I had a comprehension problem, but that was ignorance, no ill will intended. Since my accident, I have experienced only a few people who have assumed I am mentally challenged or illiterate because of my appearance.

On this first trip, I did find some stores impossible to navigate in a wheelchair. I am still not surprised to encounter such obstacles today — aisles that are too small or clothes racks that are too close together — even in our supposedly enlightened age. It doesn't bother me. I just don't go in. It's the stores' loss; they lose out on my business. Like I've said, there are more of us wheel-chair-dependent people than they probably realize. Government legislation says I must have equal access, but I don't like shopping, anyway. I'll leave that fight to someone to whom it matters.

I left the mall with mixed feelings, but overall I was happy. I'd had no major issue joining society as a disabled person; I had enjoyed myself and looked forward to my next outing.

Over at physiotherapy, things were improving but very slowly. I progressed from standing on the tilt table to standing by myself holding on to a ladder-like structure attached to the wall. Mereille placed my hands on a rung as high as she could stretch my rigid arms, then gave me a boost while holding on to my weak hands, and I was standing.

I didn't feel very confident; my knees wanted to buckle, my thighs screamed with the weight, my hamstrings cramped, my calves burned, and I held on like I was about to fall down a cliff. Mereille asked me to bend my knees, hold the position, and then stand back up again. It wasn't hard, bending; it was hard to hold it and impossible to straighten my knee. My leg shook under the strain, but with effort I slowly straightened it.

"Gooda!" shouted Mereille. "Two more!"

What seems impossible sometimes becomes possible with effort and the kind of encouragement I received from Mereille. It was never easy; advances were achieved with sweat. I didn't realize then, but this stage was easy compared with what it would be like later. Rigidity was becoming my enemy. When I tried to sit, my hips would not bend and I went down as though my back and pelvis were fused together. I could not stick my behind out, and that prevented me from sitting far back in the wheelchair, which became a major frustration because whoever was helping me had to grab my pants and pull me back, creating a tightness in my groin commonly called a wedgie. Very uncomfortable!

About this time, Mereille had me stand beside the exercise mat with my hands on a bedside table. My balance was poor. I required assistance to stand, because as soon as I put any effort into doing something, my tone kicked in, extending my back and pulling me backward. Eventually, I was able to stand with support and had gained enough strength in my legs that at the end of August, Mereille tried me with a walker.

In occupational therapy, Doreen was encouraged enough by my left-hand improvement to rig a mobile armrest and keyguard to aid me in typing at a computer. The armrest, which had the ability to swing in any direction, held my elbow because I was too weak to hold my arm up for typing. The keyguard had holes over each key so that I could move over the surface without picking up my hand or striking each letter. I took these devices home on the weekends so I could use my computer.

Around this time, Beth devised a small letter board taped to a lap pillow that enabled me to spell words by sliding my arm over the surface and pointing my finger at a letter instead of using the eye-gaze board. This made conversations much easier and less tiresome for me. I could converse using more abstract ideas and therefore explain what I was thinking in greater clarity.

Around this time, by the end of August, with the introduc-tion of the computer-assisted devices and the letter board, I considered myself no longer locked in. I could converse with most people; with the eye-gaze board, I had been limited. I had spent more than three months in that living hell we call the locked-in state. I will never forget. The lying in bed, the total dependence, the frustrations, the questions of *why me*, the unreality, the never-ending thoughts. Thinking, thinking more, forever thinking. But above it all, overriding everything, love. Love *does* conquer all. Love of God, love from family and friends, and the love Jill and I share. It may sound simplistic and corny, but it's true.

Strangers going through a similar experience have asked me, via the internet, how I got through it. I tried to think of a clever answer, something to inspire them, but I drew a blank. I could have told them clichés like, "You have to think positive," "You *will* fail if you don't try," "Think of small gains as major gains," and so on. All of them are true, but they are not my real reason for accepting and working through it. The real reason? Love. I felt love from God, from people I hardly knew, from patients, friends, my family, my children, and Jill. All we ever want — or at least all I've ever wanted in this world — is love. I felt such warmth and love from people that I was satisfied. All was okay despite every personal loss. Love empowered me to overcome any obstacle or wall in my way. Love allowed me to accept any disability that couldn't be overcome. I hope I never forget this lesson.

But I'm sure I *will* temporarily forget this lesson, as I get frustrated on a day-to-day basis. As my obsessive personality demands things be done *now*. As my children do things differently than I would have. I will be successful and happy if I can remember to stay focused on what really matters in life: love. All the rest is secondary.

I remember seeing Lou Gehrig in an old black-and-white newsreel, saying goodbye to his fans at Yankee Stadium. He knew he was dying of amyotrophic lateral sclerosis, and as his fans solemnly listened, he said, "Today, I consider myself the luckiest man on earth." Before my stroke, I thought, *How touching. What a nice thing to say in front of thousands of fans. He's telling them how much he appreciates their support.* Now, I know how he felt: he sincerely *did* consider himself the luckiest man on earth. He felt their love, and there is nothing more powerful in this world.

CHAPTER 19
SEPTEMBER

September always feels like a time of renewal. In New Brunswick, the prevailing winds switch from the south or west to the north — colder but fresher. Later in the season, the trees acknowledge this change with a spectacular splash of colour.

September produces a conflict of emotions. The smell of north in the air promises walks in the country, wearing brightly coloured sweaters, snuggling with a loved one in front of the fireplace in the evening, and the smell of fresh apples. But it also means the loss of songbirds and flowers, summer swims in the river, and drowsy late-summer afternoons.

I did not recognize the changes as intently that year because I had not experienced summer other than the heat; it was my lost summer. I got depressed if I dwelled on it, for I loved the summer: the cottage life, golf, boating, bonfires, and refreshing swims. I missed those experiences, but I chose to concentrate on the present — my goals, my rehabilitation, my progress — rather than think of the past. I had mourned everything I had missed doing that summer and tried to leave that grief behind. It was my choice: wallow in self-pity, remembering the past, or live for the present and make the best of it.

My physiatrist gave his consent to remove my antiembolic stockings because I was now moving my legs enough to prevent clots from forming. Great timing! I would have welcomed this loss a few weeks earlier, in the heat of summer. I'm being sarcastic; I was ecstatic to have them removed in any case. Now I needed to work on getting the feeding tube removed.

The feeding tube was bothering me more these days by twisting and irritating the edge of my skin where it entered my abdomen. The edge was raw and tender to the slightest touch. The junction between the peg and the IV tubing kept falling apart during feedings, creating an awful mess. I had to show Sharon I was eating enough, so I ate everything. I made sure I drank high-calorie drinks and finished all of my meals, no matter what they looked like. I coughed and choked everything down except when I saw Sharon passing by — then I suppressed any sign that I was having difficulty eating and smiled like this was no sweat.

Beth taught me the correct way to swallow. I had to keep my chin down; I choked if I looked up. My cough reflex was good, so I was not scared of aspirating food into my lungs, but choking was never fun, especially in a cafeteria full of people. A little crumb was usually the culprit of a major coughing spell. Well-meaning people rushed over to pat my back as though congratulating me on my superb choking performance. I never wanted to draw attention to myself, but I did.

I never found puréed food unpalatable. I was so glad to taste anything that I surprised myself by eating everything. Most of it didn't look appealing, but it tasted fine. However, I would not recommend puréed pancakes: they look and taste like uncooked batter. Sharon was fond of saying she could purée anything and I'm witness to the fact that she could, but was it palatable? Don't try puréed salad! Sharon made it very presentable; she even puréed a tomato, put it in a mould that looked like a tomato, and placed it on top. Disguised or not, the salad tasted like grass. When she chopped, mashed, and then puréed salad ingredients into an applesauce-like consistency, they ended up looking like mulched grass and tasted like it, too.

Other than these two minor glitches, I was surprised how good puréed food could be. My only experience with this type of food had been feeding my children when they were babies and watching my patients in hospital. It was I who often inflicted this culinary variation upon them. I cringed at the thought of ever having to eat such food and used to say to Jill, "If I get to the point that I have to eat puréed food, shoot me!" After September, I never turned my back on Jill.

My preconceived idea of what puréed food must taste like was the same as most preconceived ideas: not true. I must have eaten well enough in both quantity and quality to convince Sharon, because at the end of September, my physiatrist removed the feeding tube. Despite my eagerness to be done with it, I did not give it up easily. As he yanked to pop it out, after removing the water in the bulb that kept it in place, my stomach rose with his hand. My abdominal muscles clamped around the tube, as though angry at losing what they now considered a part of their anatomy. My physiatrist was nothing but determined; he wanted that tube despite what my abdominal muscles thought. When the spasms had calmed down, he braced his left hand against my abdomen, gripped the tube, and pulled. Every abdominal muscle, all together, in one massive, mother of all spasms, grabbed my belly into a knot like a clenched fist, and my eyes bulged out of my head like those of a squished frog. Son of a bitch, that hurt!

It took thirty minutes for my abdominal muscles to begrudgingly relax. But it was worth every minute of discomfort and spasm: I was free! No catheters or tubes. It was all up to me now — a major step toward independence. I could now breathe and eat on my own. My rehabilitation would proceed full speed ahead, with no encumbrances. Or would it?

Hope. I still had a lot of hope, but it had been four months since my stroke. My speech was a disappointment. I could make only vowel sounds: "Aaaaaa, eeeeeeee, iiiiiiii, ooooooo, uuuuuuu." I had started to eat — admittedly, food no one else would want. My left hand now moved enough to direct my power chair. I needed help to stand, but once up, I could stand under my own power. Maybe the first step in walking was around the corner. Maybe.

I continued to be tormented by the dilemma of whether, at a certain point, I should accept a disability or whether I should never accept a disability and keep fighting. It had been four months and my right arm showed very little signs of awakening. My body was rigid, fused together; my back and pelvis moved as one unit. I had very little control over my legs. Tone made them stiff, unwilling to participate in my recovery.

I reluctantly knew by this time that I would have to accept some long-term disability. Sometimes determination isn't enough; some damage can't be overcome, no matter how hard I might try. I read the statistical outcomes of brainstem stroke and knew I should be happy just being alive and no longer locked in. It isn't lack of determination that keeps some people locked in. Rather, some organic damage can't be overcome, no matter how hard they pray, exercise, or use willpower. They're just plain unlucky and have to accept their plight in life until medical science can learn how to repair the damage.

So when should we survivors of brainstem stroke pack it up, accept our disabilities, and learn to live with them? Well, it appears we can continue to show improvement over a number of years. The progress is painfully slow compared with the first six months, and you expend far more energy than the results show, but some of us improve with effort. It has to be you, or the little person inside you, your intuition, who says, "That's it. Too much energy's being wasted with not enough results. I have to get on with life, get a job, find a career, whatever."

I still had hopes for walking. I was unable to picture myself not walking. In my dreams, I walked. I felt like a walker. This fellow called Shawn, he walked. But an inner voice called to me, saying, *No, you're not. You are a wheelchair guy. You will always be a wheelchair guy.*

I tried to ignore that voice. I was unwilling to accept it. My physiatrist had told me in July that he didn't think I would learn to walk, but that didn't shake me. I'm a doctor, too, and God knows I've been wrong before. I chose to feel that he was only trying to prepare me in case I didn't learn to walk. So it was a great shock when Mereille and Doreen told me one September day that I would never walk, at least not functionally.

At home on the weekends, Jill was making plans for my eventual return. We had converted our living room into a bedroom for me, and I was sleeping there in a rented hospital bed. But it felt temporary; the piano and formal sofa and curtains constantly reminded me that this wasn't really a bedroom. I was sleeping in our living room, like an outcast. Besides, where was Jilly? I wanted her beside me. I couldn't conceive of never sleeping with her again. I still looked up the stairs at our bedroom and assumed that I would be going up those stairs someday. I had not slept with Jill in all this time. I required a nursing assistant to turn me frequently throughout the night.

I tuned out when Jill started making plans about remodelling the downstairs bathroom and making it wheelchair accessible with a cut-out vanity, raised toilet, and roll-in shower. I think it was too real, an admission of my disability. The cost of renovations worried me. I was receiving a disability cheque by this time, and it covered expenses, but that was all; any extra expense would require a loan. I didn't see how we could afford the payments of another loan. As I mentioned before, I should have talked to someone about my concerns — at least Jill.

Jill had talked to Doreen about designing the bathroom to make it appropriate for me: where to put the grab bars, what type of shower. I listened, detached, agreeing to decisions but not really believing this discussion would bear fruit. I was not helping her make decisions about renovations. Besides, fellow patients had implored me not to make any hasty changes. They had improved and now they were sorry they had gone through the expense and effort of renovating their homes. I listened to them, a part of me still holding out for that miracle.

One morning, Mereille and Doreen were working on my posture near one of the exercise mats. Jill had just spoken about the necessity of doing the renovations at this time. Doreen said, "You know, Shawn's never going to walk normally. He will never use your stairs to get up to the bathroom. He will never get up from a chair and just walk to the kitchen."

I watched Mereille's face as Doreen said this. She kept her head down and worked on my right hand, bending and massaging my stiff muscles. Doreen's face was red and her conversation hurried; she was uncomfortable having to tell us this.

My stomach tightened. Doreen's forecast and Mereille's silence told me enough. *They think I will never walk, too! It isn't just my physiatrist's opinion.*

A part of me, probably the doctor part, knew this was true. But the real me, the real Shawn, hoped for greater things. He hoped to walk out of there. He hoped to be walking the old foot path to Sand Point at his cottage. He hoped to canoe again. He hoped to walk on a beach, lie in the sun, go for a swim. He had been hoping for so many things and now those hopes all came crashing down.

I stared at them impassively and, amazingly, did not cry. I was numb, devoid of feelings, lost in my sorrow. All gone: my dreams, ambitions, and hopes.

This conversation occurred in the morning, just before lunch, so I didn't have time to recover from the emotional shock before I ventured into the cafeteria. I ordered as though nothing of any significance had just occurred, but in fact, my life had once again been turned upside down. I didn't taste the food. My mouth was dry; my throat constricted. I ate mechanically with no thought other than *No walking. They don't think I can learn. I will never walk ... never walk ... never walk ... never walk.*

Everyone else ate and conversed as usual. Again, I was reminded that life continues on. Even though a tragedy had occurred in my life, nothing had changed for anyone else in the world.

After lunch I spoke with Jill about what Doreen had said. "Waa di' you thin' of tha', waa' Doween sai'?" At this stage, I was unable to pronounce the consonants at the end of words.

"I think they said you won't walk."

"Wha di' thea saa it?"

"I don't know."

"Do you bwieve it?"

"I don't know."

I could see Jill was crushed and feeling like me. I was dependent on Doreen and Mereille and valued their opinion. I knew what they had said was true, but it took some time for me to accept it. I now had to toss away my dream of walking normally. But they didn't say I wouldn't walk at all, and over the ensuing days and weeks, Doreen and Mereille didn't stop ambulating me. In fact, they seemed to be increasing their efforts to help me walk. I had to change my ambition from walking normally to maybe — maybe someday — taking a few steps with the walker on my own. After that, who knew?

I have never completely abandoned my hopes of normal walking. Who knows what medical science may come up with? Researchers are experimenting with stem cells, and maybe someday they will be able to inject my brainstem, which will differentiate into neurons, and I'll get up from my wheelchair. *They* might. I noticed how it had changed from "*I* might" to "*they* might." I was slowly accepting that I wouldn't be able to walk no matter how hard I worked or how set my mind was. The only possible way was through a medical breakthrough. Unlikely, but still ... hope.

I had to accept so many things I would never be able to do, and I mourned each loss. For some things, I held on to the hope that someday I might be able to do them. Other things I knew I could or would one day be able to do with modification. And some things I accepted I would never be able to do. One of these things was walking on the rocks in front of our cottage.

CHAPTER 20
THE ROCKS

While I was lying in the NICU, I had thought about the possibility of never walking again. I couldn't fathom the idea of never walking on the rocks in front of our cottage on the river's shore.

Our cottage was built during the fall of 1997 at Buckleys Cove on the Kingston Peninsula, on a rocky outcrop of the Saint John River, across from the town of Grand Bay-Westfield. Our cottage bears the full brunt of storms that come from the south and build up waves through the open waters of an area of the river called Grand Bay. Conversely, the cottage is protected by the hills behind it from storms that come from the north and east, and it faces the usually mild west wind.

As a boy, I spent every summer with my grandmother and brother just two lots over from our present cottage, in my family's camp. I am grateful for the summers of my boyhood. They are happy memories: sun, swimming, boating, playing soldier with my cousin Bruce, fishing, exploring, and later, when boyhood ended, the first exciting attempts at socializing with girls.

Bruce and I fished most days when we were young. We ventured out upon the river in a rowboat, set anchor by a sunken wharf that was in front of the family cottage, and fished for perch. Occasionally, we got an eel or a bass, but most of the time we caught the iridescent green-yellow, scaly perch. We threw them back but kept count of our catch, adding up our totals throughout the summer. We discovered that the best type of lures to catch perch were the curtain hangers from Bruce's cottage. I wonder if his mother ever figured out why her curtains drooped from mysteriously missing hangers!

On sunny days, it would be too hot to fish on the river, so we went to Buckley Brook, where it was cool. We knew the best spot to dig worms, the best fishing holes, the best way to travel upstream, and where to stop so we wouldn't encounter bears. We travelled up the stream, going from fishing hole to fishing hole, struggling through bush in some areas, and jumping from rock to rock, always excited even though we had danced this dance many times before. No matter how hot the day, it was always cool down by the brook. The best fishing holes were where a small waterfall, created by the brook falling over a natural dam, made the water deep, dark, and foamy. We never fought over who got the best fishing hole. We would, without discussion, square it all up the next day. Nothing had to be said; friends are like that. We were in another world, a boy world of filtered sun, coolness, grins, laughs, and friendship.

Boys of ten would never talk of feelings or even know how to express such abstract ideas. As Bruce and I grew, our interests diversified and we spent less and less time together, but when we are together today, the bond that formed when we were ten holds fast. We intuitively know who gets the next fishing hole. There is no contest between us. No need; boyhood friends are just like that.

We always made sure we were back home by noon because the baker, milkman, or grocery man might show up on the hill, blowing his horn. There would be a treat waiting for us. The grocery man had chocolate bars or candy, the baker had chocolate patty-pans, and even the milkman had a treat: small containers of cold chocolate milk. These men probably never thought about the influence they had on our little lives, but even now when my boyhood friends and I get together, we often say, "Do you remember when the baker arrived? We'd stop what we were doing and come running, crying 'Baker! Baker!'"

In later years, Jimmy, Steve, Bruce, and I would swim, play tennis, boat, and, in the evening, load up our canoes and spend the night on deserted beaches. We took pride in our campfires, building a lean-to in case of rain, cooking our own grub, and talking like adults. These were important lessons on our road to independence, although we were just boys having fun.

We had other friends, too, like Peter, another Jim, Mike, Barry, and a few others, but they were sometimes not around, busy with their families, whereas we four were always there together for the whole summer.

As we grew older, Sand Point would become the scene of our foray into the graces of interacting with the opposite sex. Men of the campfire turned into quivering idiots when confronted by these confusing yet mysteriously appealing companions. A year before, they had been girls who were friends, and not very fun generally, but one summer, something happened. To them? To us?

The first girl who ever paid attention to me was a girl from Toronto named Jane, who was down visiting her cousin at her cottage for two weeks. I didn't know why she liked me, but I was honoured by the attention. I was always the quiet one; I existed on the periphery in my circle of friends. I preferred it that way. But she saw me there and drew me out. Two weeks flew by and, alas, my first love had to leave. I was curious about what had happened. *Why does a girl from Toronto like me?* I wondered. The girls in my class at school didn't seem to notice me. I didn't think they knew I existed. Maybe it was the new hair growing on my legs, or maybe the two or three on my chest. Or maybe it was those hormones I'd been reading about. *Whatever, maybe Linda or Pam or Barbie will notice me this year at school!* Whatever Jane had seen, Linda, Pam, and Barbie missed it. I was still invisible to them, the same ol' Shawn.

At that point, I met my first long-term girlfriend, who became my high-school sweetheart. We went out for more than three years. We should have been dating other people, but even knowing that, I probably wouldn't have changed anything. High-school sweethearts are special, sharing so many new experiences, and those years can be so dynamic and exciting.

Buckleys Cove held many memories for me, and I wanted my children to experience cottage life on the peninsula. We stayed at my family's cottage for a few summers, but I grew restless for our own place.

Our cottage is built of cedar logs, with three small bedrooms in the back and a great room that comprises our kitchen and family room. The deck is large, with an overhanging roof, and most days I can read or work on my computer there, protected from sun or rain. The cottage is close to the rocky cliff and about twenty feet from the river. As I write this story, I am sitting on the deck with the waves rolling onto the rocky cliff.

The cliffs are responsible for the constant sound of water breaking that we can hear from our cottage. I roamed these rocks in my youth, stepping out onto the old wharf at low tide, marvelling at how lichen could survive on these rocks, and watching the developing mosquito larvae in the pools formed in the crevices. Offshore, cormorants would dive for fish. An occasional loon came over from the marsh across the river, and osprey soared overhead, looking for a meal.

I sat on those rocks, years later as an adult, designing and then building a floating dock. There were many things to consider: I wanted to build it so it could be broken apart, floated over to the beach, and then hauled up by two people at the end of the season before the ice came. I also had to consider the tides (the Saint John River empties into the Bay of Fundy, which has the highest tides in the world), the winds from the south that whipped up huge waves, the decrease in the river's water level as summer progresses, and how to secure the dock to the shore. I spent time on the rocks watching the river and designing the dock in my head. When I finally had it built and in place, I forged a natural path from our cottage down the rocky cliff to the dock.

I grew up with the rocks, played on the rocks as a boy, and dreamed about and built my dock on the rocks as an adult, but now I would never walk, play, or dream on those rocks again. But really, I didn't spend *that* much time on the rocks, so why were they almost the first place I envisioned never being able to walk on again? I guess they symbolized a loss of many things to me: walking along the footpath to Sand Point, in the forest, along the stream, on the beach — all gone.

I'm back at the cottage now. Ramps have been built, the bathroom altered, poles installed for me to hang on to, but essentially it's the same. The cormorants still dive, the loons still cry, and the osprey still soar. My dock is gone, but the rocks remain, as they always will. I am happy being close to them, hearing the waves break on their face. That's good enough for me — it has to be.

CHAPTER 21
LATE SEPTEMBER

As my left arm improved, the nurses encouraged me to use it by brushing my teeth, combing my hair, and shaving. It frustrated me and there were times I felt like giving up, but something would always happen to encourage me to keep going. The nurses gave me practical advice based upon their experience, and I listened closely. They instructed me on the best underwear for men in a wheelchair. My habitual boxers don't work well in a wheelchair for someone who has to be pulled back as often as I do. But why are the flies so complicated in briefs? It's hard enough getting access standing up, but try it in a wheelchair. It took me a while to discover which brand has the easiest access. (That's my secret.)

I used a commode for the first time in September. My sitting balance had improved enough to allow me to sit on a commode with a lap belt. Simple changes like this could be surprisingly liberating.

Then came my first shower. I was wrapped in a blanket, placed on a commode, and wheeled down the corridor to the shower. Before my stroke, I took showers rather than baths, so it felt great, but the best part was that I didn't have to swing on the Hoyer lift. I felt more in control, even though I couldn't lift my arms to help with the showering. The nurses hosed me down, scrubbed me with soap, and shampooed my hair. I was quite familiar with the whole procedure; I used to do the same with my dog.

Bedtime became especially irritating to me. Since June, I had started getting prepared for bed at 9:00 p.m., because the nurses had to bathe me, brush my teeth, clean my tracheotomy tube, and start my tube feeding. This all took time, so I was resigned to starting early, but now that I was free of the trach and my tube feedings, I felt I should be allowed to stay up later. I found myself hiding like a child from the nurses to avoid my bedtime. Many of my fellow patients felt the same, and we plotted schemes to allow us to stay up later.

The nursing staff had to start getting us ready so early because they wanted all the work done before the night staff of two people came on at eleven. I realized this, but I still hated being told when to go to bed at the age of forty-seven. But it's part of institution-alized living, and I had to accept it.

I wouldn't have minded if I'd been able to read. I have always read before sleep; it has been a habit since childhood. I've always loved books. I love the feel and the smell of books. I love being taken to another world by only words. It's like dreaming, really, except that you are fully awake and someone you don't even know is directing the scene. I think it's interesting how a person who wrote fifty years ago can direct that scene for me now.

I listened to audiobooks, which were fine, but they weren't the same. I watched TV, but it didn't fill the void. I was lost when they put me to bed early. I watched ball games until the sleeping pills took effect.

One day, I was finally able to turn a newspaper page. It was difficult, especially to get the paper to lie down flat, but I did it.

Turning the pages gradually became easier, and eventually I could read a book in bed with a laptop table that my cousin Lynne had given me. There were many frustrations — pages not staying put after I turned them; my fingers accidentally turning more than one page at a time; the whole book sliding off my lap table to the floor — but it was worth it. I was reading.

I read hardcover books. Paperbacks were much too difficult with one hand. At first, I read stories by stroke survivors, especially by brainstem stroke survivors, but I also read fiction. One of the first books I read was probably symbolic: *Going Inside* by Alan S. Kesselheim. It was a memoir about the experiences the author and his wife shared canoeing along a northern Canadian river and then holding over for a winter up there. I thoroughly enjoyed the escape of being transported to a wilderness freedom I might never be able to experience again.

I was reading; there was no need to hide from the nurses any longer.

I am lucky I enjoy reading, for as the saying goes, you can never be bored, if you are a reader. And I have time to read with this condition. And read. And read …

I mentioned that in June, the Saint John Medical Society had held a benefit dance in my honour. Well, they made a video of the event, including personal get-well wishes to me from the people who attended. One weekend when I was home in late September, the physician most responsible for organizing the affair and a pharmaceutical representative visited me to show me the video. I was still emotionally labile and cried in front of them during the part where friends were privately sending me their wonderful words of love and encouragement. Those sincere, generous words touched my soul. I felt like Tom Sawyer witnessing his own funeral.

I now also had a bushel basket full of letters and cards from my patients, which also made me cry every time I started to read them. I had to take a break after reading only a few. People were sabotaging my fight to gain emotional control by being so caring!

Other people were generous in other ways. One of my patients, who taught Transcendental Meditation (TM), offered to teach me the method in September. When I was still working, I had expressed interest in learning about TM but had never found the time. He came to my home one weekend and taught Jill and me the method. After a few weekends of instruction, the end of the teaching was marked by a ceremony. Unfortunately, my emotional lability was on full display as I roared with laughter while he carried out this traditional symbolic ceremony that included flowers, ordinary household items, and incense. I pinched myself to stop laughing; I tried thinking sombre thoughts; I tried to remove myself from this scene. Nothing helped. It wasn't at all funny, but in that state, whenever I found something the least bit happy or different, I exaggerated that joyful emotion by breaking into loud gales of laughter. Likewise, when anything was the least bit sad, I cried. This emotional instability continued to plague and embarrass me.

I dared not go to a comedy or sad movie in a theatre. One night, Pierre, the brain trauma victim I had once mistaken as "not right in the head," and I went to the same movie. Pierre had a funny sense of humour, and I spent many an hour laughing in Stan Cassidy over something he had said, so when he started to laugh about something during the movie — which wasn't a comedy — just hearing him laugh made me laugh. Soon both of us were laughing uncontrollably in the packed theatre. I imagined people thought this paralyzed, emotionally uncontrolled man must be simple, and this thought only made me laugh more over the absurdity of the moment.

However, the emotional lability wasn't funny: It made me feel like an inadequate, incomplete, less-than-human being. While laughing during the ceremony at home or in the movie theatre, I prayed, *Please, God, help me stop this. I do not find this funny. Please help me stop!*

I hoped TM would tranquilize my soul and help me gain control over my emotions. It is supposed to be practised before breakfast and supper, for twenty minutes. I couldn't ask the nurses to get me up before the morning shift came on duty, so I asked them to awaken me to meditate in bed. Not a great idea, because I quickly fell back asleep. Then, when I would try to do the second TM of the day before suppertime, I was so tired from my therapies that I fell asleep once again. If the object of TM was to relax me, I suppose it did work!

I eventually found that I couldn't practise meditation with drugs onboard and in an institution. I had expected meditation or mindfulness would be valuable tools for relaxing and increasing energy and happiness, and I regretted I couldn't continue.

I could have used energy, inner peace, or whatever it took, because on the ward I learned firsthand what constipation felt like. All my life I'd had a bowel movement daily; I had never had a reason to think about it. I treated patients who complained of constipation, as it was a daily complaint in the hospital, brought about by sudden inactivity. I must admit, though, I thought the nurses were all anally fixated. Often the first thing they related to me in the morning was who "had gone" and who hadn't. I prescribed medication without giving much thought to what the patient must be going through.

Payback! I found out why the bowel movement is the holy grail of hospitalized patients. It isn't fun being constipated. I was sorry I had been so indifferent about it with my patients. I will spare you, the reader, the details but suffice it to say, twenty years later the struggle continues. But what goes in has to come out. I'm testing that theory.

Speech lessons continued to be tedious. Twice a day, I worked to regain that which I had lost. It seemed to me then that a big part of who I was left along with my voice. That's not actually true, but at the time I mourned that loss. My voice still existed in its former intonation on the telephone: "You have reached the home of Jill and Shawn Jennings. We are not at home. Please leave a message after the beep. Thank you." And on a few tapes from when I had recorded myself singing and playing the guitar. I had to remind myself that I was still me, regardless of what my voice sounded like. It wasn't strange listening to my past voice, nor did it make me melancholy. I focused on the present and refused to dwell on the past.

I must have taxed Beth's patience, because as she tried to get me to say *moo*, I broke into laughter. I felt so embarrassed by my apparent hilarity over her lessons. I apologized to her every time, even though I knew she understood.

Actually, it was quite sad; I had a hard time saying *moo*. I would joke around and tell everyone, through my letter board, that Beth was trying to make me sound like a cow, but underneath that humour I was quite anxious. I didn't have enough breath support to say a few words, such as they were. And my pronunciation was extremely poor. People had a hard time making out anything I said, although I sounded understandable to my ear. I was shocked when Beth recorded me. It made me realize that I presented, to those who didn't know me, a far different person from who I was or what I thought I sounded like.

During speech lessons, Beth had me begin with a consonant and add all the vowels: for example, *maa, mee, mii, moo, muu*, or *saa, see, sii, soo, suu.* Each word, each sound, was a battle, but it was only the beginning. Those sounds that used the middle of the tongue, like *m*, were easier. More frustrating were soft sounds, like *h*, and sounds made with the front part of the mouth, like *v* or *f*, or the back of the tongue, like *k* or *g*. I couldn't pronounce the end of words. When I tried to say "What are you doing tonight?" the words would come out slurred together as "Whaa r ya doin' tani?"

I was more tired after speech than I ever was after physio or occupational therapy. The amount of energy I used to say simple phrases for a half hour far exceeded the results. Part of this energy was wasted, because a lot of the air came out of my nose. My soft palate was paralyzed, so it dangled down the back of my throat like a dead fish. When speaking, the palate is supposed to close, sealing the nasal passages and thereby allowing all the air to come out of your mouth to be used for speech. A good portion of my air — and I didn't have a lot to begin with — came out of my nose, leaving only a small amount for speech. My breathing muscles were paralyzed; the muscles required to move my vocal cords were spastic. It all seemed too much at times, but Beth always encouraged me, and I was making small gains. I tried to give it my full effort despite the failures and I still do. I do stomach crunches, I work on word inflection in sentences, and I breathe into a spirometer daily for more breath support. Nothing comes spontaneously; nothing comes quickly, without effort, but it does improve for some brainstem stroke victims. I have been so fortunate to get some function back. I don't forget that and I try harder tomorrow.

Trying harder — that's tricky for us with rigidity and tone. The harder I tried to do something like bend my hip, the higher the tone in the muscle became and the harder it was to bend my hip. It was a classic Catch-22. Sometimes I could use tone to my advantage such as in standing, but don't ask me to move from that spot.

Mereille *did* ask me to move from that spot. I had been standing with a table in front of me while I put pressure on my hands. This was to reduce tone in my legs and arms. Doreen always came to work with Mereille, and together they had been addressing my posture (sitting and standing) and balance. I couldn't perform the acts of sit-to-stand, stand-to-sit, lie-to-sit, or rolling over. I was stiff; my pelvis and back acted as one. "Bend at the waist, Shawn! Bend those hips!" Doreen and Mereille would cry. My muscles, because of the tone, would not let go.

Standing is a good way to relieve tone, so Doreen and Mereille had me do this often throughout the sessions, but the day came when they asked for more: stepping. I was excited. This was what I wanted to do. *Now we're cooking!*

Excitement soon turned to frustration as my legs showed no desire to move. I needed help. Mereille steadied me from the back, correcting my posture, gait, and pelvic movement. Doreen stabilized my walker and hand control, while Betty or Jill moved my feet. My entourage and I must have been a curious sight as we moved down the gym.

I knew that if I was to walk, it wouldn't happen today or tomorrow, but I grew disappointed at my lack of progress. Mereille and Doreen didn't stop, however. They faithfully took me on a walk every day; despite telling me I would not walk normally, they hadn't given up. This gave me hope for some type of walking.

It was hard to watch others progress. Other stroke survivors started walking, but they had all had the one-sided or cerebral type of stroke. I had no other brainstem stroke survivors to relate to, so I watched the others. I was happy for them as they progressed from immobility to walker with assistance, then to walker alone, then quad canes, regular canes, and finally, walking alone. I was well aware that I was different and that I couldn't compare my stroke to theirs, but I couldn't help it.

I *was* happy for their improvement, but there was a part of me that cried, *Why? Oh, why can't that be me? Just one step, or any significant improvement to be happy about.* I was envious; I wanted a eureka moment. I couldn't believe how calm everyone was, accepting their improvements as though it was a natural course of events. They worked hard for what they gained and I suppose to them it seemed slow, but I felt that I was working hard, too, and I deserved some reward.

I was unique around here, but I started to feel more akin to the patients with quadriplegia. I suppose it's natural that we tend to seek out people in our society who are similar to us, and I was paralyzed in all four limbs like they were, only from a stroke rather than trauma. I shared some of the same problems they had, and they could do some tasks better than I could and some not as well.

There was a big difference, though: I had a chance to improve over a few years, while they could improve only to a point and then they would have to await a medical breakthrough. I realized I had little to complain about as I watched Amanda and Todd, and other patients, struggle.

Amanda was a single mother in her twenties who had arrived at Stan Cassidy during the summer. Her daughter, Mackenzie, was about a year old and quickly became the darling of Stan Cassidy. Amanda had broken her neck when an all-terrain vehicle had flipped on a short ride up a hill from a party to her car. That short ride changed her life forever. It is difficult to accept that sometimes a simple mistake or accident can change a life so drastically or result in death when at other times, the same incident might cause nothing but a chuckle or a sigh of relief. Amanda's passenger was not hurt, but she was left quadriplegic for life.

Amanda had bright eyes and a cheery disposition despite her circumstances. It was impossible not to like her; she did not hide her emotions and had no pretense around others for the sake of propriety. She tried to control her life, and this resulted in frustrations, angry outbursts, and, on more than one occasion, a slammed-down phone. Yet Amanda was tender and giving in spirit. I couldn't smile, talk, or gesture in any manner to make conversation, yet she always included me in her conversations: "Isn't that right, Shawn?" "What do you think, Shawn?"

She was a buzz saw of activity and emotions, undoubtedly resulting from her medications and circumstances, but I suspect that underneath she had probably been quite a bubbly young lady before her accident. She flew around Stan Cassidy in her power chair at one speed: fast. She twirled in circles; the chair became an extension of her persona. As she watched TV, she moved her wheelchair, turning one way or another, always on the move, as though the chair were a part of her hyperactivity. This was a young woman with things to do, adventures to experience, and loves to explore.

My heart went out to her. She will never know the influence she had on my emotional recovery. How could I feel sorry for myself when Amanda faced far worse prospects of recovery than I did? Oh, Amanda wasn't always brave, nor did she even try to be stoic, but Amanda was real. She didn't try to hide behind some romantic ideal of how a heroic quadriplegic should act; she would have laughed at that. No, Amanda lived in the present tense. It wasn't pretty; it wasn't fun. There was not a damn romantic thing about it, but it was her reality.

Maybe Amanda was a big crybaby when interacting with her doctor and nurses, or maybe she was brave all the time — I don't know. But I do know Amanda was real, and I thank her for being her.

Todd became my friend, my roommate, and, in a way, an inspiration as well. Todd became quadriplegic in his early twenties, in a motor vehicle accident late one night, driving home from some event. He hadn't been drinking but he was tired. That would be his mistake, for he fell asleep, and when he woke up, he was lying in a ditch unable to move. He is quadriplegic for life, unless, hopefully, a medical breakthrough is made.

Todd had already been at Stan Cassidy for a few months when I arrived. He had red·hair and a round, cheerful face. I imagined him as a child, energetic, impish, an I-never-took-to-schoolin' type of guy, a regular Huck Finn. He reinforced my impressions with the stories he told me of adventures that had happened in his youth, of life in rural New Brunswick and in small towns, of his loves. Rural life trivia I learned from him: "Ever eat squirrel? Not bad. I wouldn't eat skunk, though."

Todd never talked a lot, but he was the first fellow patient to talk to me for any length of time. He made no assumptions about my abilities and spoke to me as though I was mentally competent, unlike a lot of people when they first encountered me. Most impressive of all his qualities, he always tried to understand me, despite my speech impediment, and he never said, "Oh, is that so?" as people often did when they couldn't be bothered to try to decipher my speech or were too frustrated or embarrassed by it. I understood why people got exasperated and embarrassed trying to comprehend me; *I* got frustrated trying to be understood. But Todd never appeared to. He and Jill comprehended my speech better than even I did. *How did he get that?* I would wonder. *I didn't even understand what I said.*

Todd and I laughed. We laughed about situations we got into, our conditions, stories we shared, jokes, and typical dumb, male humour.

Todd loved country music and always had the country channel on TV. I liked rock, folk, jazz, New Age — almost any type of music, with country music on the low end of the scale. We had many good-natured laughs over this, and he showed me the value of this music form (not to mention the pretty women in country music!). I told him he had been sent to torture me with his brand of music.

Todd was human, and although he put up a brave front, especially during the day, I often heard him struggle with emotions at night. He fought with the bed sheets, trying to turn; his remote might fall just beyond his grasp; his bladder might spontaneously empty; the pain from his muscle spasms might be tormenting him. And besides the physical distress, I couldn't imagine the emotional turmoil that my friend must have been going through.

I had been able to experience true love and the thrill of watching my three children grow. I had felt the joy of coming home from work and having kids rush to me with unconditional love. I had had a productive and fulfilling work life. Although these things were still obtainable for my friend, I knew that they would be a struggle for him. I didn't know if he knew that life still goes on for the disabled. I thought he might be thinking that his life had stopped, that he would never find a job, hunt again, or find someone to love.

I heard him cry softly during the night sometimes. It might have been with pain, frustration, or emotional turmoil; I never questioned him. I think he would have been uncomfortable discussing emotions, so as the day dawned, we moved on and forgot our demons of the night.

Todd struggled hard to do things on his own and became as independent as he could, and in doing so he gained my admiration. Like Amanda, he demonstrated to me how fortunate I was. I couldn't feel sorry for myself while these two young people were struggling bravely for some form of independence. I thank Todd for becoming my friend, and although he didn't intend it, he, too, became instrumental in my emotional recovery.

So as September ended, I was slowly climbing out of my diving bell, as Jean-Dominique Bauby called being locked in in his memoir, *The Diving Bell and the Butterfly*. It was ironic that I should be locked in, for loss of control had always been the ultimate expression of a phobia that had affected me for years.

CHAPTER 22
THE IRONIC

Locked in. As I said, it was ironic that I should have this condition, and I was reminded of this as I slowly emerged from my cocoon. In the past, I've had an irrational fear of not being in control or of not being able to leave a crowd when I needed to. If there was any situation I was not in control of, it was being locked in. Every body movement or function, except for my eye movement, was in the control of someone else. Someone wiped my nose and my bum, fed me, made me defecate, turned me in bed. I was dependent upon others for every aspect of living. This was the epitome of what I had always feared.

I think I suffered from social phobia (the fear of social situations) and perhaps emetophobia (the fear of vomiting). I say "I think" because I have never seen a psychologist, probably owing to denial. It was too embarrassing for me to talk about. People with social phobia often fear being humiliated in front of others, so they try to avoid those situations. A lot of people with social phobia go untreated and live on the outside of society, mostly unseen, because even the act of going to a doctor or psychologist to talk about their symptoms is humiliating and hence triggers the phobia and anxiety. Another Catch-22.

I didn't dwell on the diagnosis too much — I just knew I was phobic about something. In fact, for most of my life, and still at the time of writing the first edition of *Locked In Locked Out,* I thought I was battling agoraphobia. But upon reflection, after the book was written, I became sure it wasn't that phobia. Agoraphobia is a fear of wide-open spaces; I loved the outdoors, alone or with people.

When I was in my twenties, I was having a few beers with a friend of mine when he admitted he sometimes feared being in a crowd and called it agoraphobia. I responded to his admission by telling him that I experienced a similar anxiety. And so, I privately adopted that as an underlying, not fully expressed diagnosis and dealt with the symptoms, until my reflection after writing the first edition of this book.

The irrational fear of not having control over a situation, combined with my fear of vomiting, produced anxiety in certain situations. I felt the need to be able to leave anywhere I was, such as a plane, a restaurant, a lineup, the passenger seat of a car, or even a barber's chair, without causing a commotion. I feared vomiting or fainting in front of everyone, thereby bringing attention to myself. But if I drove the car or sat at the end of an aisle, I felt fine. (The same would perhaps be true if I controlled the plane, but the plane's passengers would require professional help!) It seems so foolish to me now, but most phobias are, like being afraid of a little mouse that wouldn't hurt anyone.

The fears probably started when I began university, but they didn't become fully developed until I was in my early twenties. My first full-blown panic attack happened while I was eating supper at my girlfriend's home. Her family was large, with eight siblings, and we were all sitting around the dining table when I

suddenly felt hot, then nauseated, followed by sweating and nervousness. I thought I was about to pass out. I never told anyone;
I just quietly stopped eating and hung on. I know now that it was
a panic attack, but at the time I had no idea.

I made excuses, thinking I must be suffering from hypoglyce-
mia or ulcers or, later on, with my new but green medical wisdom,
dumping syndrome. I denied the truth. I think I knew quite early
what was wrong. *Shawnie boy, you are bonkers!* I couldn't accept it.
I was not alone in this; most people would rather have something
physically wrong with them than accept a mental problem.

The phobia got worse. In movie theatres, I had to be in an
aisle seat; if I went to a restaurant, I had to be near the exit; line-
ups bothered me; and air travel became a major anxiety. In some
of these situations, the major angst occurred before I actually
had the experience. This is called anticipatory anxiety, and it can
lead to avoidance behaviour. Panic attacks are not pleasant, and
I became fearful of the fear. I eventually knew what they were,
but knowing didn't help. The attacks made me feel worse than
anything I ever experienced from my stroke. Probably the worst
thing about a panic attack is that nothing does happen; you survive to have another attack without any intervention, and no one
has any idea of what you just went through.

My panic disorder went on for years, and then it started
happening in the office. In the morning and at noon, my subconscious mind became aware that I was stuck there for hours. I
couldn't get out without going past all my waiting patients. I was
trapped, not in control. As silly as it sounds, I panicked before
my office hours began, in the morning and at noon. Once I was
under way, I relaxed.

Repeated exposure was not working; my phobias were
not getting better. I read books on the subject and even coun-
selled patients with similar problems, often referring them to

psychiatrists or psychologists. "Now, now," I'd say when they were dismayed about being referred to a mental health specialist. "You're not crazy. The brain gets sick like any other organ. It just gets sick differently. Society has a poor attitude about mental illness. You shouldn't think of yourself as weak."

How hypocritical! I was keeping my dirty secret to myself. Jill was the only one who knew, and I don't think I was completely honest with her about the extent of my phobias. I needed to tell my own family doctor or refer myself to a psychiatrist or psychologist, but I felt embarrassed about having a phobia over such silliness; it lowered my self-esteem. I chose to accept it and put up with it, but it made my life miserable.

The panic attacks were so devastating they left me weak, quiet, a pitiful character, really. I felt inferior for being unable to beat this thing. It was selfish of me to not seek help, because I was less than I could have been for Jill. I was stuck by being too proud to seek help. Foolish man! I was choosing to make my life miserable.

However, a wonderful thing happened in my midthirties: I became depressed. I'm being sarcastic, because depression was anything but wonderful. It was like a big, black pit I would never find my way out of. It was cold and lonely in there. I could share the feelings of panic with Jill, but there was no way to share depression, nor would I have wanted to. I was on my own, and this time I knew I couldn't live with it; I had to turn to someone for help.

The depression started with a decrease in appetite, especially in the morning. My appetite improved as the day wore on, and by bedtime I was ravenous. Then my sleep became disturbed. I usually fell asleep fine, exhausted by the stress of the day, but within a few hours, I awoke for a night of tossing and turning. I felt agitated the longer I lay awake, and when it was time to get up, I struggled, feeling anything but refreshed. My mood became depressed in the morning but improved by the evening. I felt my ability to concentrate at work slipping, my mind wandering as my patients told me of their symptoms. I lost weight, and tiredness set in, a fatigue that left my legs trembling with any exertion.

Clinically, I was curious to be experiencing these symptoms. Depression was one of the most common illnesses I saw. A day as a family doctor did not go by without diagnosing a new case or following up with a depressed patient. Now I was that patient.

Patients had not exaggerated the fatigue experienced in depression. I was amazed at how physically tired depression made me feel. I was confronted with these symptoms each day, and a part of me was fascinated to experience them. But the depressed mood state, the variation in my mood over the course of the day, the sleep disturbance, the appetite disturbance, and the lack of concentration were plain for me to see. I couldn't deny it: I was depressed.

I suppose the experience of being depressed helped me later to accept my stroke — why not me? There were probably a number of events that led to this depression. This is true for most cases of depression. Usually, we can't pinpoint a single event that led to it. It does happen; sometimes grief over a lost loved one can go on too long and lead to depression, but usually that type of depression is reactive and is best handled with supportive psychotherapy. A clinical depression results from depletion or imbalance of neurotransmitters. My imbalance of neurotransmitters probably resulted from a number of factors. We do not yet understand how life events and our reactions to them result in physical changes in the chemicals of the brain.

My underlying phobias no doubt played a major role in becoming ill — the old noggin had had enough. Also, at that time I was facing a number of stresses. I was under some financial strain because a group of physicians and I were establishing a medical clinic, a number of my patients had become ill from a flu shot administered at my office a few months before, and a patient who was not much older than me and with whom I had grown close had recently died from a blood problem.

Dave was a very pleasant chap who suffered from a type of phobia and I, of course, related to him. When he developed hypoprothrombinemia, an inability of the bone marrow to produce platelets, we had no hematologist in Saint John, so I sent him to Halifax for treatment. After he had been in hospital there for a few months, they sent him back to me, resigned that all active treatment attempts had failed.

Things were going downhill, and I continued to be solely responsible for him. I phoned the hematologist in Halifax regularly and followed his directions, but to no avail. Dave's platelet count remained dangerously low. One night, he had a brain hemorrhage in his sleep and died. I had expected this could happen at any time, but I had also hoped for a miracle, that one morning I would walk into my office and find his platelet count had risen significantly. That's the damn thing about hypoprothrombinemia: occasionally, the bone marrow suddenly starts working and the platelet count rises.

I felt so sad for Dave. He had kept a graph of his platelet count on the hospital room wall, plotting it every day. He would be encouraged by a small rise that I knew was not significant, even when I told him so, and I couldn't dash his hopes altogether. He never let me talk to him or his family about what could happen, because he wanted no negativity. That was fine, but I felt his family was ill prepared for what did occur.

I found looking after Dave very stressful, and with the added stresses of the flu vaccine, financial challenges, and my phobias, I became depressed a few months after Dave's death.

Jill couldn't believe I was depressed. A little down, maybe, but not depressed. The psychiatrist, likewise, was surprised. I hadn't seem depressed when he had seen me around, but when I explained my symptoms to him, he agreed that I was suffering from a depression.

I said the depression was a wonderful thing to happen to me, and it was. It finally prompted me to see a psychiatrist and reveal that I suffered from a panic disorder. Just being able to tell somebody about my phobia was a relief but also, in taking my history, he found reasons that might have made me prone to developing these phobias. It was like someone turned on a light in some dark tunnel in my brain. Why hadn't I thought of this? Of course! I received cognitive therapy and it helped greatly in my recovery, but explaining why I suffered from this fear did not cure my problem — I wish it were that easy.

My psychiatrist prescribed an antidepressant drug that worked like a charm on my depression, and as an added benefit, it also blocked my panic attacks. Within two weeks my depression was lifting and by four weeks, it was nearly resolved. Treatment for depression often has to continue for six months, assuming there are no setbacks.

Meanwhile, my panic attacks were being blocked. I found I could go into restaurants and not worry — I enjoyed myself. I could sit in the middle of a row or travel on planes without panic. With the drugs blocking the anxiety, my brain soon learned that there was nothing to fear in these situations. Phobias are often caused by events or fears that start in our childhood. The light that was turned on for me, through the psychiatrist's probing, involved my parent's divorce.

I was six years old when my parents broke up and my mother, brother, and I went to live with my maternal grandparents. I didn't see my father much after this, even though he still lived in the city. The psychiatrist asked me what I felt about my dad.

"Nothing," I replied.

But over the following days, I realized I must have felt something. Yes, I had felt abandoned. He had been a good father. I remember sitting on his lap as he sang and rocked me to sleep, playing with him on the beach, sitting in the tub while he bathed me. Now he was choosing not to take me out or have anything to do with me. I must have been hurt.

It was a different time in the late 1950s, and fathers didn't have the privileges they do now, but I think I would have maintained contact more than he did — just a short visit on my birthday and at Christmas. My mother didn't want him in our lives at all, but that shouldn't have stopped him. If I had been him, I would have fought her in court to be able to see my child. I learned that my mom forgave him alimony payments for the sake of leaving us alone. So he chose money over me? I'm sure that wasn't true. My father and I started to forge a new relationship when I began an independent life with my own family. I found him to be quite a nice guy. He was in the process of moving back to the Saint John area from Saskatchewan upon his retirement when he suddenly died.

In the last few years, I've searched my family tree, and I found an interesting detail about my father. His mother died in childbirth when he was eight years old, and he and his brother were sent to an orphanage and lived there for many years because their father couldn't look after two young boys by himself. That must have been very traumatic for my father — far worse than my situation. Perhaps my father found the loss of his two boys, who were near the same age he was when he lost his mother, too psychologically threatening. Did it reawaken old fears for him? Was visiting us too painful for him, even unconsciously?

About a year after the divorce, my mother suddenly left for Montreal and left my younger brother and me with our grandmother. This was what might have caused psychological trauma. There is nothing more psychologically threatening to a child than being abandoned by parents. It's an ingrained fear, a situation that threatens survival for the young in nature. Many studies have shown how the breakdown of the parental bond can lead to psychological disorders for the child, which can be permanent without intervention. I was surprised to learn, about ten years ago, that Mom had been gone for only six months; as a child it had seemed like years. My gran was a wonderful lady, but she wasn't my mother. So within a year, both of my parents *chose* — as I saw it from a child's perspective — to leave me, and I was scared, hurt, and confused.

I know my mom would never intentionally hurt me, and if she had known leaving might inflict psychological harm upon her children, she wouldn't have gone. Perhaps she thought she was so mentally distraught after the divorce that she was unfit to be a mother and we were better off with our grandmother. I wasn't angry at Mom when this revelation came to me as the psychiatrist probed my psyche, but I was disappointed in her lack of insight or maternal instinct at the time. How could she have left me and my less-than-two-year-old brother?

Emetophobia may have been forged during the time Mom was gone. That was the last time I vomited. I must have had the stomach flu, as we called it then, and I distinctly remember lying on the sofa in my grandmother's living room after vomiting, feeling very miserable and wanting my mom or dad. Again, I'm sure my gran was great, but she wasn't my parent, and I felt the need for parental comfort. Now, does the act of vomiting unconsciously re-create that painful scene? Does my psyche do everything in its power to protect itself from a painful memory, even overriding the natural process of vomiting? I'm not sure, but I get very anxious when I am nauseated, and, until my stroke, I hadn't vomited since.

I never talked to Mom about this; it would have served no purpose and would only make her feel guilty and miserable. I'm sure she had a very good reason to leave, and it was probably painful for her, too. In the 1950s, child psychology was in its infancy. I'm sure the notion that her boy would perceive the separation as abandonment never entered her head. As an adult, I can understand and forgive, but little Shawn didn't understand — in his mind, his mom and dad didn't want him.

I have always been dismayed and saddened by the long-term effects that childhood trauma can have on a child's personality and life. I have witnessed this in my practice, and I'm sure what I have seen is only the tip of the iceberg. Most children experience far worse things than I did, but even a short breakdown in the parental bond can lead to lifelong anxieties unless addressed.

Maybe all of the psychoanalysis I went through with my psychiatrist had no relevance in pinpointing the cause of my phobias and anxieties, but it seems likely that they arose from the need to control my own well-being and not be dependent on anyone else.

Now that I was not experiencing panic and anxiety, I felt, for the first time in a long time, that I was in charge, and that transformed my life. So the depression, in a way, was a blessing, and it caused another change in my thinking as a doctor. Before this, I had never given psychotherapy much credit; I had thought the best cure for mind disorders was medication. After my experience, I saw the value and need for therapy in my practice, and I referred patients to psychotherapists earlier and more often than I had in the past.

I also started to delve into the past more with my patients who were suffering from neurosis. I started booking a long therapy session for patients I perceived as needing insight. I grew to love this time, but in a busy practice it was difficult to fit in this type of session during the day. So I saw these patients as the last appointment for the day, and that worked well. I was amazed at the wealth of information I obtained, but whether it was worth the effort in view of the results is questionable. But people enjoyed the opportunity to talk. I think, most of all, they perceived that someone cared, or at least I hoped they did.

Depression changed my life for the better; I loved living. I think it made me a better doctor, and it again reinforced to me that something positive could come from a negative thing. I'm hoping and trying to make positive things happen from this stroke. I've enjoyed life to the fullest since my depression, and I'm not stopping just because I've had a stroke.

So you see how ironic it was that I was locked in. It was perhaps a control phobic's nightmare, and I lived through it without a panic attack. It was as if I had been prepared.

CHAPTER 23
OCTOBER

I didn't require as much care now that my feeding tube and trach were gone, and that meant I no longer warranted a private room. My first roommate was ideal for my transition. His name was Colin; he was about my age, friendly, but quiet. He had suffered the rupture of a brain aneurysm and was making significant progress in his rehabilitation: walking, using one arm, and talking. However, his thinking process was disordered and he had expressive aphasia, which meant he couldn't find the right words to express his thoughts. We were quite the pair: he couldn't express and I couldn't physically say what we wanted to convey to each other. It was amazing that sometimes we did actually manage to understand each other, but most of the time we gave up trying, shrugged our shoulders in defeat, and laughed.

Colin lived in Fredericton, so he went home a lot, leaving me with the room to myself. It was similar to my previous room: one large wall of windows, the rest of the walls of white-cement brick, a closet, and a bathroom. The only differences were that there were now two beds instead of one and I now shared the small, ancient bathroom with two people in the adjacent room. My window looked out onto a small parking lot, seldom used, in the back of the building. A basketball net sat silently in the yard, awaiting a patient who could use it to explore their capabilities, but I never saw that happen.

Stan Cassidy's inadequacies as the major rehabilitation centre for New Brunswick became more apparent to me. *How dare they treat people with life-changing disabilities this way?* I must admit, I had never thought much about rehabilitation when I was actively working. Rehabilitative medicine has always been the poor sibling in terms of medical funding, but that was no excuse for providing disabled people with a facility that had inadequate-sized rooms. Disabled people have always had to fight for their rights: access to all public places, cutaway curbs, public transportation, parking places, and an array of other issues. It looked like this was a similar situation: the government would continue to provide an inadequate rehabilitative facility unless the disabled population or their supporters protested. However, I was quite comfortable there, and I didn't hate Stan Cassidy; the attitude and atmosphere were a credit to all the staff, from the director to the janitorial crew. I just wished there were a modern facility with larger patient rooms to enable easier nursing bed care and to help patient morale.

By October, my sliding board was gone forever. With help, I could pivot from my bed to a chair using a walker. I couldn't stand up or sit independently, but I was happy without my board — it was more progress.

At physiotherapy, they started to use a LiteGait, a type of treadmill. I was suspended from above by straps that were tied around my waist and groin. The treadmill was supposed to signal to my brain the normal pattern of walking while taking away gravity. The signals weren't getting through for me. The strong tone in my legs never decreased and my knees and hips continued to refuse to bend. In fact, the LiteGait made the tone worse; I needed gravity — weight on my feet — to reduce the tone.

Doreen tried everything to facilitate my sit-to-stand, but she couldn't break the tone in my back. Likewise, the muscle tone prevented me from rolling over in bed, which we practised repeatedly. My body remained as stiff and straight as a board, and effort only increased that tone.

Tone continued to plague me even in speech. My facial muscles were tight, and even when I did manage to break the tone and move my lips a little, my spastic laryngeal muscles produced only a small squeak of a voice.

My left arm and hand continued to improve, and I could now shave with an electric razor (incurring a lot of facial burn) and brush my teeth (dripping toothpaste down my arm and on my pants), but my right arm and hand remained very spastic and immobile. Up until this time, I had hoped my right arm was just months behind my left, but that looked more and more unlikely. With the improvements to my left arm, I graduated from arm control to hand control of my wheelchair and was now able to travel with little effort. After I had achieved this, I thought that maybe if we transferred the hand controls to the right side, that would force my right hand to work. Doreen agreed to let me try. It was very frustrating, and after a few weeks of trying, I gave up and went back to my left-hand controls with relief.

I continued to go home every weekend, which made staying at Stan Cassidy bearable; it gave me something to look forward to. I went home on Friday afternoon and returned Sunday night, thereby spending only four nights a week at the centre. Jill was the reason I was able to do this, because I needed a lot of help to do even the most basic of activities, like standing, sitting, and eating.

It is a shame that insurance companies make life so hard for disabled people. They always request documentation from professionals *at the patient's expense* and hold up payment or authorization until they receive it. A disabled person, especially one who is newly disabled, is having a hard enough time dealing with this life change without having to worry about money and care. It is a cruel endeavour and so unnecessary. I understand that insurance companies are subject to many cases of fraud, but assuming every case may be fraudulent is wrong. I know that by being vigilant, the insurance companies are keeping our premiums lower — or are they keeping their profits higher?

In my case, I was tetraplegic, meaning four of my limbs were paralyzed. (*Quadriplegia* is the most familiar term for paralysis in all four limbs, but the term is reserved for the condition that results from spinal cord trauma.) It would have taken only an insurance company representative coming to see me to determine that I couldn't stand or use my arms and that my wife couldn't possibly look after me twenty-four hours a day. These companies should assume the client, especially one with a major illness, is telling the truth. If they won't make the effort to see for themselves, they shouldn't wait for letters from the occupational therapist, physiotherapist, physician, and whoever else, or stop payment until all documents have been received. I am fortunate to have enough resources to be able to withstand these lulls, but others may not be so lucky.

I saw many cases of this while working as a family physician. There were a few cases of insurance abuse by clients (and I tried to point them out to the insurance company), but there were many more cases of abuse generated by insurance companies. People pay high premiums for many years and when tragedy does strike, the insurance companies should show more compassion than they exhibit now.

My disability insurance company was fine — they caused no problem at all — but my health insurance company was stubborn. This type of treatment did not surprise me in the least. I told Jill to comply with their requests, no matter how silly they might seem, and not to take it personally. But Jill had not been conditioned to this type of treatment and found it stressful, tiring, and frustrating to have to obtain all the requested documentation. The caregiver, already burdened by what is perhaps a new role in the relationship and new responsibilities and tasks, is now asked to be responsible for compiling information — and it better be timely and correct or they won't pay. Insurance companies should give caregivers a break and be responsible for getting the information from professionals instead of burdening the client.

At this point, we were encountering no major obstacles from the insurance companies, and renovations to our home were proceeding on schedule. The little talk I had received from Doreen and Mereille helped me to accept that my life was never going to be the same. I was not going to walk upstairs to the bathroom, so if I was going to stay home, I had better make the downstairs completely accessible. Concern about cost continued to nag me in the back of my mind, but it had to be done. Jill handled the details of what to buy — the type of shower, toilet, cut-out vanity, and so on — and I watched her in awe.

I felt hunger for the first time since my stroke. I was now eating without any extra liquid supplementation. I dreamed of a thick, juicy steak, but I didn't have the ability to chew so I had to be content with puréed food. I was happy just eating, and hunger felt good — a return of a normal sensation.

At home, the computer enabled me to contact the outside world. I continued to speak to friends via email, visit disability sites, and exchange ideas with stroke survivors. My left arm improved enough so that we could remove the armrest, I could use the computer mouse instead of the keyboard cursor, and I no longer needed a key guard.

I still felt restless at times in my wheelchair and experienced compulsive urges to get out of it and onto a chair. However, these feelings of agitation were fading, and I was becoming more accustomed to my seat. My feelings of confinement, restriction, or entrapment in my chair were melting as my bum toughened and I accepted the facts. *You are effectively a paraplegic, buckaroo! Oh, maybe you'll fool them and walk — DON'T GIVE UP! But here and now, you're in a wheelchair.* A few months before, I had thought there was no way I'd get used to a wheelchair, but I did. I had no option.

In Fredericton, I went to my first movie; in Saint John, I went to my first hockey game. Patti, my nursing friend who had done so much, accompanied us. I enjoy watching hockey: the speed, the flow of the game, the formation of play patterns, the defensive strategy, and the charged atmosphere in a close game.

I grew up playing hockey on backyard rinks and on the street. My friends and I didn't play organized hockey outside of school — why, I'm not sure — but we played a lot. Like most Canadian boys, I endured frozen toes and the painful thawing process more than I care to remember. We never became really good hockey players, but we didn't care; among ourselves we had great games. We were Jean Béliveau, Bobby Hull, Norm Ullman, Alex Delvecchio, Dave Keon, or Gordie Howe. The sounds and exhilaration of the game have never left me: skates crunching on ice, the chase for the puck, the perfect pass to someone in flight, and, of course, the triumph of picking the upper left corner of the net and the darn puck actually going there — the perfect goal.

I was never a good hockey player, probably because I had no natural talent (although I won't admit that to my kids) and I never had any formal coaching or skills practice, but I loved the game. I gave up playing around the time I entered high school. I was thin and the only way to survive on the ice if you have no bulk is to be fast, and I wasn't that, either. After getting banged around quite a bit one night, I gave up the game, but not my enthusiasm.

I was thrilled to be back in the rink, watching the Saint John Flames, a minor professional team. Four months before, I could barely raise my thumb and I had watched the Stanley Cup playoffs with disinterest on TV, but now I was back in Harbour Station, the arena in Saint John — another milestone mark on my way back to normalcy. Many friends and patients came to greet and wish me well; they seemed happy to see me out in public, but no one was happier than I was.

They say life is often reflected in the games we play, but maybe sometimes the games we play reflect or predict our lives. When I was a child, my friends Allan and Ronnie and I would watch *Western Theatre* on Saturday afternoons. CBC was the only channel we could get, so we didn't have much of a choice. Black-and-white thrillers of cowboys, "Indians," rustlers, and no-good, gosh-darn varmints. It fed our eager imaginations and after the show, we would meet in back of Al's house to act out our own tales.

Al's father owned a black car trailer that doubled as our stage-coach. We had six-guns in leather holsters strapped to our legs by pieces of rawhide. My guns had silver barrels with Western designs etched along their length and white handles engraved with horse heads. The handles were actually plastic, but I imagined they were carved ivory. I had no idea what ivory actually was, but I once heard a cowboy on TV remark to another cowboy that his gun was carved from pure ivory and the other cowboy seemed impressed. We could use blast-cap strips — if we had them — and that was way cool, but unnecessary for the plot. A "bang-bang" did nicely, and we loved making the ricochet sound.

Al usually set the scene and Ronnie and I added suggestions. In fact, we often got so carried away with the suggestions, we'd forget the premise and have to start all over again.

We were often riding the stagecoach into Dodge, carrying gold or a lovely young lady, the general's daughter, when no-good bandits would come out of the woods to steal our precious cargo.

"There's one, Al! To your left," I shouted.

He fired and the varmint fell from his horse.

"One's hopped onto the stagecoach!"

Ronnie struggled with him in hand-to-hand combat, nearly falling out of the stagecoach a couple of times, but each time managing to force his way back up.

Suddenly, I was in trouble: a bad hombre had managed to climb onto the stagecoach from behind me and had me by the throat. I fought hard, but he had me good.

"Al!" I yelled, motioning that I was being strangled.

Al was driving the stagecoach but he pulled off an incredible feat: he managed to wrap the reins around one leg, stand up, turn around, and bash my assailant over the head with his gun. No wonder we loved this guy as our director.

"Thanks, partner."

Al shrugged it off like it was another day's work — no big deal.

Meanwhile, Ron had gotten rid of his bad dude by flipping him over his back, onto a stump that was sticking up as our stagecoach drove by. We had seen a similar scenario on a trading card. There was a series depicting the Civil War that was popular at the time, and one card showed someone — maybe Stonewall Jackson — being thrown off his horse and getting impaled on wooden spears that had been driven into the ground for this purpose. Way too cool! We couldn't pass up the opportunity to incorporate this move into our play. A bad dude always got impaled somewhere along the way.

We continued shooting until, invariably, Ronnie got shot. He went down with great fanfare, clutching his chest, grunting, then falling over the side in a fantastic tumble routine. I suspect Ronnie got shot first because he would rather have been playing cars. Cars were his passion throughout his life.

This was the clue for my eventual demise. However, I was not so eager to end our little play, and I liked to play the struggling hero who got shot and told his pal to leave him.

"I'm shot, Al!" I grabbed my chest and fell to my knees.

Al glanced back. We had outdistanced the bandits, and they had fallen on Ron and were now taking his boots. An unlikely plot, I know, but cowboys always seemed to be trying on dead men's boots (and they always fit!) — and besides, we were only six years old.

Al lifted me down from the stagecoach and cradled me on the ground. "Hurt bad, partner?" he asked.

"Reck'n I'm not gonna make it, Al."

"Hush now. We gonna gets you a doc and gets you all fixed up like, once we gets you into town."

"No, Al, I've had the biscuit," — big cough here, blood coming up — "but you got to do me a favour. Leave me here."

"No way! I'll —"

"Listen to me, dagnabbit! I can't go on … I'm gonna die. But Al, listen to me." I grabbed his shirt and pulled him toward me. My voice was becoming shallower and I was panting between each word. "Ya gotta save the pretty miss from those bandits."

"I'm not abandoning you. You're like a brother to me."

Ronnie was getting a tad fed up by this point, and he ruined our scene by saying, "Come on, guys!"

"Shut up!" we both yelled.

"Ya gotta do me this one favour. Gimme a gun and I'll hold 'em off."

"No!"

"I want to die fighting. You wouldn't deny a dying man his last request, would you, Al?"

Al pulled out his gun and gave it to me. He climbed up onto the stagecoach, and with a "Giddy-up!" he drove away.

I lay waiting. As the bandits approached me, I killed a few. But the rest of the gang pumped a few more bullets into me and I died. The music swelled as the camera pulled away from the scene.

Al always seemed to get the girl, but it didn't matter; I got to play the hero and Ronnie got off early to play cars. We played many variations of this, but Ronnie always seemed willing to get knocked off early and I loved being disabled by bullets. Often, I was shot up bad but managed to stagger back to town, falling in a heap as the townspeople rushed to my side.

Years later, Ronnie died in a snowmobile accident. He was in his early forties. At the age of forty-five, I had a stroke and became disabled. Al's had a tough life; he's had to dodge a lot of bullets, but he's still riding.

I'm going to play the other scene, Al; I'm getting to Dodge, shot up but staggering into town.

I guess my sex life has been healthy, or whatever *healthy* means in that context. Oh, I know, it means doing whatever both partners are comfortable with. But *healthy* does sound rather odd when used to describe sex, doesn't it? It isn't like a healthy habit we try to adopt, such as eating green vegetables to prevent cancer or quitting smoking or cutting down on fats or exercising (well, maybe it could be considered exercise). I've never heard of anyone prescribing sex twice a week for a patient's health, although I can think of a few who might benefit.

Understandably, I did not think about sex once from May to October. I don't remember a dream, thought, or fantasy of any type. I was now into my fifth month and I had not experienced an erection, not even an early-morning erection, signalling pee time. As this was the area of my anatomy the nurses often tackled first as they washed me, I was always afraid they might find "Henry" rising up to say hello (a friendly fellow, but sometimes quite inappropriate). Thankfully it never happened, but I grew curious about his non-appearance. I knew strokes had no bearing on the ability to have an erection — which proves it doesn't take brains ... oh, never mind. Nor was the absence of an erection a recorded side effect of the drug I was taking. Maybe it was psychological, but then why was there no early-morning erection?

Experiencing some kind of mild sexual dysfunction is common after a stroke: premature ejaculation, erectile dysfunction, performance anxiety, fear of causing another stroke, a myriad of problems. I knew all this, but I could think of no reason for erectile dysfunction. I was more academically interested than worried as to the cause.

Sam was a pretty, young nurse who always appeared cheerful, confident, and friendly, although she later admitted to me that she had been rather wary of me because I was a doctor. One night, Sam showered me. Usually the nursing assistants do this task, but that night she had to do the chore. After my shower, Sam wheeled me back to my bathroom to dry me. As she rubbed my feet with a towel, a peculiar sensation came over me, and I thought I was about to urinate. In a panic, I tried to warn Sam that I suddenly needed to pee, when to my utter amazement, right out of the blue, I ejaculated onto my thigh. Luckily, a towel was covering my genitals. I had had no warning, no erection — nothing! My body went through powerful spasms of orgasm, my bottom slid out of the chair, my feet flew up in the air, and I groaned.

"What was that?" Sam said.

"Spa-spa-spa-spasm," I tried to say.

"I've never seen you get a spasm like that."

"Twi-twi-twi-twice a wee.'"

"Are you okay?"

"I'll be fi-fi-fi-fi'e."

Sam went back to drying my feet while I panicked. A smell pervaded the small washroom. At first, I didn't recognize the odour, but soon I remembered.

Oh no! Does she know what happened? Should I tell her?

I think Sam had an idea of what had happened, because she slowly rose up, looking like she was struggling with what she was about to say, as I was.

Then Bessie walked in. She was an older nurse and I just about died.

Oh Lord, how does this look? A middle-aged old goat with a pretty, young nurse and the smell of sex in the air!

There *is* no God, because if there were, I wouldn't be alive right now — sudden death was the only solution. I did what I always did when confronted with a personal dilemma or crisis like this: nothing. I froze. My mind went catatonic. Vapours of burnt wires drifted up from my head. Overload! Overload!

There are some things a man can explain, but sitting in a room with a pretty, young nurse with ejaculate on your thigh isn't one of them. This was one of those no-win situations, like when your wife asks you if she looks overweight. I was dead, dead, dead.

I think Bessie thought Sam was taking too long, because she took over my care and prepared me for bed, leaving Sam to clean up the room. Bessie reached to take away the towel that was covering my genitals. Ejaculate exposed! I quickly pretended my thigh was excruciatingly itchy and rubbed it madly with the towel, letting it "accidently" fall to the floor after what I discerned was a reasonable amount of time for scratching without raising suspicion. I prayed I had successfully removed the evidence. *Yes!*

While Bessie put me in my pyjamas, I noticed Sam picking up the towel and taking it away. *Is she holding it differently? Out to her side? Does she know? Or is it my imagination?*

I couldn't get to sleep; my embarrassment over what had just occurred was tormenting me. And *what* had just happened? I hadn't been fantasizing about Sam and she hadn't done anything improper. It had been a normal day and a normal shower — nothing unusual. I thought this probably wouldn't have occurred with Denis or Nadir, two male nurses (or at least I hope it wouldn't have happened, or I would have been even more embarrassed). I don't have a foot fetish that I'm aware of. What had happened?

I experienced another episode of spontaneous ejaculation without an erection a short time later. On that occasion, the nurse was simply rubbing my sore shoulder when suddenly, without warning, I ejaculated. Again, completely non-sexual — my wife and two of my children were in the room with the nurse and me. Talk about your wires being crossed!

I seemed to be super-sensitive to any sensory stimulation at the time. I have subsequently researched this to see if spontaneous ejaculation is a known side effect of brainstem stroke or of the antispasmodic medication I was on, but I couldn't find any literature on the subject. Probably my fellow spontaneous ejaculators are also too embarrassed to mention it! But don't be afraid to give me a hug if you see me. It has never happened again.

I saw the humour in the whole scenario after I got over the acute embarrassment. *My friends will enjoy this story,* I thought.

But the humour was followed by sadness. I still hadn't had an erection, and this experience only heightened my anxiety. I loved Jill so much and it made me sad to think my sex life was over at the age of forty-six.

Why do I even mention this episode? At risk of embarrassing myself, I want to point out that I, a doctor who supposedly should know better, was anxious about my sex life after a stroke. It is very common for stroke survivors to be anxious about this, but it's often an unspoken fear, so it is imperative that a doctor or nurse bring up the subject, even if the patient seems reluctant. This is especially true for brainstem stroke survivors, who usually have more neurological deficits.

A nurse at Stan Cassidy had indirectly been bringing up the subject with me on my return from weekends at home by asking me, with an impish grin, if I had gotten "lucky." She always laughed when she said this, but even by joking about sex, she was giving me the signal that having sex was expected and normal. But I couldn't talk to her or anyone about my erection problem; I felt too embarrassed.

When Jill came in the day after the first ejaculation episode, I told her what had happened. I was not apprehensive about telling her. I was confident in our love and I knew she would take it as she did: she laughed. I told her about my anxiety about making love. It was the first time I had brought up the subject.

I sometimes went down to Jill's apartment in the evening to break the monotony. We took the Handi-Bus or, on a nice evening, she wheeled me down. In that apartment, about two weeks after my embarrassing episode with Sam, Jill and I made love for the first time since my stroke.

We both cried after. I experienced a mixture of spontaneous and conflicting emotions. I cried because I loved her so; I cried because she was so familiar; I cried because this lovemaking was so unfamiliar; I cried because my arms were useless; I cried because this wasn't our home; I cried because I could see the full moon out the window above my head; I cried because I was finally snuggling with Jill like old times.

Colin became a day patient, living at home and coming in daily for therapy. Instead of giving me a new roommate, the staff switched people to different rooms and I ended up in a ward. The ward was long and narrow, with four beds arranged side by side like an army barracks, except with less room. I resided at the end of the row, against the wall.

There were only two other patients besides me in the ward during my stay there. We had all suffered strokes and I, at the age of forty-six, was the oldest. Strokes are usually thought of as a disease of the elderly, but our room proved that impression wrong. Strokes are certainly more common in the elderly, but they do happen in younger people.

Doug was in his late twenties. He had been involved in a motor vehicle accident and had sustained some broken bones and contusions, but nothing life-threatening. A few months after the accident, he suffered a cerebral stroke. He had regained his ability to walk and speak, but was working on strengthening his gait and his affected arm.

Jim was in his late thirties and had also suffered a cerebral stroke. He had all the major chemical and genetic risk factors for stroke, but he didn't have the habits that would increase his risk of stroke; he was very active and not overweight. Jim walked and talked well and was working on the same goals as Doug.

They were both excellent fellows. We respected each other's personal space, were quiet when we perceived the need, and laughed a lot. Doug was thoughtful and quiet — I think he missed his wife and baby a lot. Jim was more talkative; he had the bed beside me and was a great help to me. He loved the Boston Red Sox, so he and I often watched the ball games on TV while we fell asleep.

Being on a ward did not change the nursing routine: up at 7:15 a.m., breakfast at 8:00, therapy starting at 9:00, lunch at noon, therapy resuming at 1:00 p.m., therapy finishing around 3:00 or 4:00, supper at 4:45, to bed by 10:00 (if they could find us). One day I got a break from that routine when a student nurse was assigned to me. She was very pleasant, and I enjoyed her company as she stayed by my side throughout the day. After a few days, she had to ask me a series of questions, and I'm afraid I might have caused her some distress. One of the questions was "What do you miss most while you're here?"

The answer was easy, but I burst out crying: "My kids!"

Most of the time, I tried not to think about them. Colin being so responsible and kind, looking after his younger sisters. Beth was cooking the meals and doing well in grade twelve — an exciting yet important time of her life — and I wasn't there to help her. And Tara, in grade eight, continued her excellence in school and activity in sports, with little guidance from us. They could give me no greater gift than demonstrating that we had raised them to be responsible and independent.

Still, I cried as I said goodbye to them after each weekend. I missed the idle chatter over meals, the laughter, and the bond of a family together. I hated thinking of them arising each morning on their own, making breakfast, going to school. They had ample opportunity to skip school, but they never did. They could have skipped studying in the evenings, but their marks showed they didn't. I was so proud of them, but I missed them so. I let my emotions go in front of this student nurse, who must have felt terrible for causing me pain. I had thought I was gaining control of my emotions, but the tears would not stop, no matter how hard I willed them to cease.

I grew tired of my disobedient emotions; I grew tired of the nursing routine; I grew tired of Stan Cassidy. I knew I had to stay to improve, so I never seriously considered quitting, but I started to get an inkling that progress was slowing down. November and December would prove to be a major turning point in my life.

CHAPTER 24
NOVEMBER TO DECEMBER: THE UNEXPECTED

Mereille tried to induce functional responses in my legs by using different exercises. I walked on stairs, on treadmills, with splints, without splints. I had electric myographic stimulation to my muscles. I visualized myself walking; *Nice and easy, Shawn. It's a nice day and I'm walking on a beach. My legs are relaxed.* The results were always the same: my tone didn't allow my muscles to relax.

Mereille always remained optimistic and encouraged me, but I could feel the change in my body. Up until then, my body had gained spontaneous return of movements; or with hard work, my function had improved. Now I was spinning my wheels. I wasn't getting the same results, no matter how hard I worked.

Before, I had felt like my body was thawing out. Each day, a new part of my body worked better than it had the day or week before. Now my body seemed frozen, with no more improvement.

The implications were devastating. I'd had hope. I had crawled out of being locked in. I was standing with a walker. I was using my left arm to eat and brush my teeth. *I can't stop here!*

I thought. *Don't leave me here. Please, don't be that cruel. Please!* I couldn't help but implore God not to let my progress stop, but to give me the strength and spirit to continue. I didn't want to think negatively, but it got harder not to. It felt like the window for improvement had closed. It had been six months since my stroke, so maybe I had to accept my current condition. Was this the improvement plateau they talk about?

Again, I was facing the old problem of when to accept and when to keep fighting. I told myself, *If I give up, I will never improve. Never. Never. Never. That is a certainty. But if I keep trying and try not to be discouraged, I have a chance. I'll keep praying for strength to continue on. But I'll do it — I will walk someday. If God will help me not to get discouraged, I will do the rest!*

So, I came to believe that my progress had slowed down but was not finished. It was discouraging to think that my rapid improvement phase had ended and this was as far as I had advanced. It was a disappointment, but it was not the end of my journey out of the tunnel.

I didn't want to give in, and with my new attitude, I wanted to go the extra mile. I wanted to fight, never give in! I balked when Doreen approached me about ordering my own power chair; I didn't want to surrender the possibility of someday wheeling my own chair. I thought if I was forced to use my right arm to wheel, it would improve.

The tone in my right hand prevented me from opening my grip, so once my hand was on the wheel, it wouldn't let go. My chest muscles wanted to pull my arm into my chest. They didn't like to relax and let my arm extend outward to the wheel.

I think Doreen knew I was wrong, but to her credit, she saw I was adamant and helped me choose a manual chair. When it arrived, a few weeks later, I was determined to use only this chair from now on. I pivoted in and tried to wheel down the corridor.

I went maybe a foot. My right hand refused to let go and, in the end, Doreen wheeled me back to my room.

I tried to use my manual chair and forsake the power chair, but I wasn't making it to my therapies. Someone always had to come and rescue me. Eventually, I gave up trying the manual chair during the day and went back to my power chair. But in the evenings, Jill helped me practise up and down the corridor. My right hand remained balled up in a fist, my skin chafed, and blisters formed on my thumb. Night after night we practised, but the tone never relented. I was wrong — I found out that you don't always get rewarded for effort. Sometimes the physical limitation is too great. That was the hard truth. But if you hit a wall, back up and go another way.

I did no better with my speech. My palate continued to be stubborn and did not close when I tried to speak. My facial muscles and tongue wouldn't co-operate, and my breath support was minimal. I wasn't laughing any longer during my lessons; either I had more control over my emotions or I didn't find anything to laugh about. I expected fast results. I had wanted to talk normally by now. I got frustrated.

At the end of October, the clocks were turned back an hour to standard time, making the evenings darker — and longer. I grew bored.

I thought I might be discharged because of my lack of progress. I was ready for the big conference someday soon, and the news that I would have to leave. I had to agree with them. The news would not be unexpected.

I was used to encountering the unexpected. In many of my previous romantic relationships, I hadn't seen the end coming, and I should have. My stroke was unexpected, but by that time, the unexpected had become ... well ... expected.

In 1979, I started my family practice in Saint John. On the second day after I opened up my door to patients, a gentleman came in complaining of a sore neck. After examining his neck, I felt he had probably strained a muscle or ligament, so I prescribed heat, exercises, and a mild painkiller.

The next day or the day after, he returned complaining that his neck muscles felt weak. He could hardly hold his neck up by the evening. I wondered if it could be myasthenia gravis, a serious neuromuscular disease. *No,* I thought. *I've just started. It's only my first week!* I was afraid I was overdiagnosing, reading too much into the symptoms. If I were wrong, it would take a long time to live it down among my peers. *You know that new doc — what's his name? Jennings? That's it. Well, he calls me the other day. He's been in practice, what, three days, and he's got this guy with a sore neck, and guess what he thinks he has. Myasthenia gravis! Ha-ha-ha!*

I asked my patient to come back the next day for a recheck. I was uneasy.

The next day, he had a new and more ominous complaint. "You know, last night, not only did my neck muscles get weak but I had a hard time closing my eyes."

That did it! Egg on my face or not, I had to get this fellow into hospital under a specialist.

I introduced myself to the specialist and explained why I wanted him to see my patient, saying that he probably needed admission that day. With skepticism in his voice, he answered with a drawn-out "Yeees?" But when he heard my patient's complaints, he was most accommodating and agreed to meet him at the hospital later that day.

None too soon, for that same night the patient had a myasthenia crisis; he stopped breathing and had to be intubated and put on a respirator. That gentleman eventually recovered and his condition remained well controlled. He lived many years before passing away from heart disease.

I never saw another case of myasthenia gravis in the next twenty years. What were the odds of me encountering this disease in the first week of starting my practice? That was just a warm-up for the unexpected.

I expected terminal diseases in my patients — everybody has to die of something — but it was always unexpected when it happened to *my* patient, someone who had become more than a patient, a friend. It was impossible to treat Mrs. Nicholson for fifteen years and not become her friend, making it shocking and unexpected when I diagnosed a terminal disease.

Medicine is fraught with unexpected diseases. They are the rule more than the exception. The most unexpected event that happened to me came when least expected and it resulted in the most grief.

The flu vaccination has reduced disease. It is especially valuable for the elderly and anyone with a chronic illness. I was convinced of its benefit and therefore strongly advised it for my geriatric and chronically ill patients. I also got the vaccine personally and had not experienced influenza for a number of years, despite my repeated exposure to the virus.

Each year, nearly four hundred of my patients wished to receive the vaccine. I administered the vaccines on two or three specific days — flu days, we called them. My nurse and I spent the whole day giving flu shots and not seeing any booked patients.

On this day, my nurse drew up the first ten injections, put five in my room, and we started. We worked hard throughout the whole day; I occasionally stopped when I had to see a patient who had come in that day for another illness, but for the most part, nothing unusual occurred.

The following evening, a Friday, I received a disturbing call from the emergency physician, informing me that Mrs. Davis had just been admitted to the ICU in septic shock. The arm in which she'd received the flu injection was grossly swollen and red. I felt my stomach twist into a knot.

When I saw her, she was in a coma and her kidneys had shut down — renal failure. This occurs when the blood pressure falls so low there is not enough force to supply the kidney with blood. Mrs. Davis's kidney had been bombarded with too many toxins from the infection. The doctors, uncertain of what pathogen was causing this massive infection, were giving her a combination of antibiotics.

I felt terrible. Her arm was obviously the site of the primary infection. It was swollen and red from her shoulder to her fingertips. The injection had to be the source. How did we contaminate a needle? And with what? My worst nightmare was coming true: I was the cause of a patient's illness and possibly her death. I had violated one of the principles of the Hippocratic Oath: first do no harm. My face and manner probably betrayed the guilt I felt, but the worst was yet to come.

A few hours later, I was paged to call the emergency department. The physician on duty asked me, "What were you using as a needle for those flu shots you gave?"

I thought he was joking, so I answered with a nervous wisecrack, but he wasn't being funny. Two more of my patients were in the ER with swollen, red arms from the injections. They were not nearly as toxic as Mrs. Davis, but after we had consulted with specialists, they were admitted under my care with IV penicillin.

I was not on call that Saturday, but I stayed in the hospital as more of my patients rolled in. My anxiety level increased with each one. *We injected more than four hundred people!* I admitted five people that day with cellulitis, a skin infection, of the arm.

I got very little sleep that night as thoughts pressured my brain: *How many patients have been affected? How did it happen?* I went over and over our procedure in the office. *Am I using the right antibiotic? What if a patient ignores the symptoms, thinking it's just a reaction from the flu shot, and seeks help too late?* I knew what I had to do: call every patient. I would check everyone's arm, even if they had only a minor mark.

The next day, Sunday, I started calling patients from the master list. Thankfully, Leah, my receptionist, was always thorough and had kept a schedule of when each patient came in. I spent the day on the phone, checking some of the patients in my office, running up to the hospital to admit more people, and checking those admitted. In the end, eight patients were admitted under my care, one who lived in Fredericton was admitted up there, and Mrs. Davis was in the ICU, making a total of ten people. It could have been worse.

By Sunday, I had found the common denominator in those infected: they had been the first ten injected the day they came in. My nurse had drawn up the first ten needles from one vial of vaccine. She gave five and I gave five. Therefore, the problem was not the way we injected. Either contamination had occurred when my nurse drew up the needles or the vial had been contaminated to begin with.

It would have been difficult for her to contaminate ten needles or syringes, especially because the procedure is to swab the top of the vial with alcohol before withdrawing the vaccine. This technique is used thousands of times every day and is pretty foolproof. No, my suspicion was the vial.

At that time, vials of flu vaccine, each enough for ten injections, came with a metal flip-top. When it was pulled off, the rubber top on the vial was exposed. It seemed to me that a defect in the rubber top might have occurred, exposing the vaccine to possible contamination. Or — a long shot — someone could have maliciously injected the vial without removing the metal flip-top. However, the vaccine is immersed in a preservative that prevents the possibility of contamination, making this unlikely. The vial had been discarded, so unfortunately we could never verify my theory.

The public health officer in Saint John at the time was great in helping me track down where this infection could have come from. Sadly, a few years later, this doctor died in a motor vehicle accident in Nova Scotia. Eventually, the chief medical health officer of New Brunswick became involved, and then the national public health office in Ottawa. They investigated my office, our procedures, and the trail of the vaccine, but no definite conclusions were reached.

All my patients recovered. The bacterium was found to be streptococcus, a very common bacterium that is often the cause of sore throats, but occasionally causes very nasty infections when introduced into the skin. The penicillin IV worked, but I had many anxious days watching as the line of red and swollen skin stopped advancing and slowly receded.

Mrs. Davis lived, but at a price. For maybe two days she had no urinary output, and then, when all seemed hopeless, her kidneys started to function. She continued to make progress and gave me great hope. However, when she regained consciousness, she was deaf. She had lost her hearing from the high-dose antibiotic they gave her when she first came into the hospital. At high doses, that particular antibiotic is toxic to the acoustic nerve, and because she'd had no urinary output to flush out the drug, the antibiotic stayed in her system too long and at too high a level.

I have been humbled by medicine many times in my twenty years of practice, but never as much as I was during this event. It was a very stressful time for me, but I was pleased I handled it as well as I did. However, six months later, and soon after Dave died of low platelets, my depression began. Whatever defences I used to deal with stress finally snapped.

When I had this stroke, I did cry to God, "Why me?" But that didn't last long — I was used to the unexpected.

CHAPTER 25
NOVEMBER TO DECEMBER: HUMOUR

My dog, Jenny, was not doing well. She wasn't eating and was getting thinner. After a couple of weeks, it was apparent to us that Jenny was very sick. Jill took her to the vet, who found her dehydrated with elevated liver enzymes and admitted her into the animal hospital for IV hydration. I felt useless during this time; I couldn't comfort Jenny or take her to the veterinarian myself. Animals instinctively choose the strongest as their leader with good reason; Jenny knew I would be of no use to her in time of crisis, and I proved her instinct right.

Eventually, Jenny journeyed to the Atlantic Veterinary College, where they did a liver biopsy and diagnosed a type of hepatitis. She recovered after taking steroids for a period of time.

Friends and family continued to provide me with support and encouragement, and I returned the favour by being a great form of entertainment. At the dinner table, I provided comic relief between courses as I regurgitated food through my nose. Not only was there a lot of space in my nose to accomplish this feat, but, because of my incompetent palate and rough swallowing ability, the food could travel up into my nose from the back of my mouth just as easily as it could go down my esophagus. My kids have seen it all: spaghetti, tuna, soup, vegetables, and other foodstuffs appearing from my nose. Colin and Beth were usually grossed out, but Tara found it hilarious. The more she laughed, the worse I laughed, making the scene quite ridiculous: spaghetti (or worse) hanging out my nose while we all hooted and couldn't stop.

My startle response created more hilarity. It is a primitive response that resides in the brainstem, and mine was damaged. You've probably seen this response in babies when they are startled by a noise. This is a common complaint among brainstem stroke survivors: sudden, unexpected noises produce violent movements in our limbs and body — movements we couldn't possibly achieve voluntarily. Jenny warned the family when someone was approaching an outside door by barking. Once, when I was sitting in my chair having a thickened drink (the thickening agent made fluids easier to swallow), Jenny yelped as someone opened the door. The sticky drink flew out of my hand and all over the room, me, the person next to me, and the Christmas tree. My mother once unexpectedly came to the door, and I threw my coffee — not hot, thankfully — into Jill's face.

We laughed about my voice; we laughed about Jill showing me how to walk (it looked like a Nazi goose step); we laughed about Jenny ignoring me no matter what I did to please her; we laughed about my attempts to sit, stand, walk; we laughed about my laugh; we laughed a lot. It was why I liked being home. My family helped me forget the pain of failure. We didn't intentionally say, "Let's not be gloomy about Dad's misfortune; let's be positive." It just happened naturally, I hope as a result of our shared family spirit.

Sometimes we have a choice: we can continue to feel miserable or we can make the effort to be happy. And sometimes it does take deliberate work. It can be easy to wallow in self-pity. You have to take charge and *choose* to live happily instead of sadly. I didn't have to choose to be happy; my family made that choice for me.

Humour has always been an important way for me to stay positive. I wasn't naturally funny. I could never tell a joke but I appreciated humour, and it is much easier being pleasant than serious. We used humour to our advantage in our family, and I used it in my practice, especially with children. Children are special. They have an inner happiness, and I loved being around them to catch just a bit of their joy. I do miss my child patients. And sometimes I didn't have to find humour; it found me.

Early in their careers, doctors tend to do everything by the book, so much so that they sometimes overdo it. Generally, this is a good practice for young doctors to engage in until they have gained experience and wise critical thinking to prevent errors. I was certainly green and played everything by the rules as they were taught to me. One of these rules was explaining to patients the procedures I was about to perform on them. But perhaps I went into too much detail sometimes and confused the poor folks.

When I had to do a breast exam on a new patient, it was my habit to explain how I would be doing it. These were the days before mammography, when the yearly breast examination was the only screening procedure available. Routinely, I said, "Now, I wish to do a breast exam today. I want you to remove your bra, then I'll have you put your arms over your head while I observe the symmetry of your breasts, looking for lumps and bumps. Then I'll have you lie down, and I'll make sure I can't feel any lumps or bumps." Kind of a mouthful, and after a while, my brain got lazy. It started to take shortcuts, not thinking about what was being said. That could get me into trouble.

One day, an elderly lady came in for a checkup, and I noticed she was due for a breast exam. I had never seen this lady before, so I started my little spiel about how I would be performing the breast exam, but I must have been tired or in a hurry, because I missed a vital part of my speech. I said, "Now, I wish to do a breast exam today. I want you to remove your bra, put *it* over your head while I observe the symmetry of your breasts ..." I left the room and went to talk to another patient while she undressed.

On my return — yep, you guessed it — there sat a woman looking like a demented Mickey Mouse, bra cups resting on her head, pointing straight up in the air.

I realized immediately what I had said, and, embarrassed for her, discreetly removed the bra from her head and proceeded with my examination as though nothing unusual had transpired. Later, after all my patients for the day had been seen and I was sitting in my office by myself, busily doing paperwork, the image hit me again. I howled with laughter at the absurdity of the moment and imagined her evaluation of my performance with her friends over tea some afternoon: *You know that new doctor, the one who took over for Dr. Grant? What's his name? Jennings? Yes, that's it. Well, he has the strangest ideas ...*

This story was funny only in that scene, not ultimately. It was sad, really, because it was my first suspicion that this dear soul was in the early stages of dementia. But funny things can happen even when people are dying of a terminal disease, and my patients and I have had chuckles in the palliative care unit. I got to know the lady, and we did share a laugh over this incident before her mind started to fail.

Years ago, I had a young female patient who had a very irritating problem: bad-smelling vaginal discharge. I tried different creams and lotions. I resorted to treating her for infections I didn't see, like candidiasis and trichomoniasis; I cultured; I sent her to specialists. She kept coming back. Everything I prescribed failed; every culture was negative; every specialist's idea failed — they and I were stumped. I was frustrated. I had known this patient since she was young, and I knew she wasn't exaggerating her symptoms. She had a very embarrassing problem, although when I and the gynecologists examined her, none of us noticed any abnormal aroma.

Every visit was the same and I ran out of ideas, but one day she came in quite cheerful. It was time for her routine Pap smear. She didn't say anything about her vaginal discharge, but the temptation was too great; I had to ask her about the problem.

"Oh, thanks for asking, but it seems to have gone away. About a week ago. I don't know how. Nothing I did."

I had hoped for a sudden cure, that it would vanish as quickly and as mysteriously as it had come. I commenced the pelvic exam by introducing the speculum into her vagina. I opened it up slowly, and there, to my astonishment, was a huge wad of pink chewing gum lying under her cervix, at the top of the vagina.

The speculum shook as I tried not to laugh. I asked my nurse for the long forceps and I quietly removed the prize. Unmistakable — it was Dubble Bubble; I remembered that smell from childhood.

I was too embarrassed for her to mention my find. What advantage would there be in telling her? Anyway, I had a new cure for malodorous vaginal discharge: Dubble Bubble.

How the chewing gum got there, I was never brave enough to ask. The truth was probably not nearly as interesting as my imagination. I've heard of putting your chewing gum on the bedpost overnight, but never …

I don't want to make a mockery of this young woman's complaint because it could have become a serious social problem for her. The gynecologists and I had ruled out any serious problem, but we didn't fix the symptom, and to her the condition was significant. It didn't matter if the odour she perceived was a variation of normal, a minor imbalance of the normal bacteria/fungal ratio, or a psychological condition; for her it was a real concern that could have led to sexual dysfunction. I'm happy to report somehow the condition resolved and she never complained of the odour again.

Mark had venereal warts on his penis. I think he was rather proud of them — a badge of male bravado — although really the warts are more like a badge of recklessness. These warts are sexually transmitted and are easily prevented by wearing a condom. It irritated me, because no matter how hard I preached to my young patients about using condoms until they were married, or how often they heard the message in school or via the media, they still came in with sexually transmitted diseases and unwanted pregnancies. Venereal warts are serious because the virus that causes them is also responsible for the development of cervical cancer. Despite saying all this, I have to laugh when I remember Mark.

I often used electrodesiccation to remove warts from the penis. This method involved burning the warts with an electrical spark after numbing underneath each wart with lidocaine.

Mark was confident and lay back with his arms behind his head as I busily removed the warts from his penis. Most men assumed a defensive, apprehensive posture, which would be expected when someone had needles and electrical instruments around their genitals, but not Mark.

"Tell me, Doc," he said, "is that your Mercedes out front?"

"No, Mark, that belongs to the cardiologist beside me," I replied.

"Well, is that your BMW?"

"No, that belongs to the other cardiologist beside me. I own the grey little Ford out there."

Mark pondered this information for a while and then said, "Not much money in dink warts, eh, Doc!"

These stories are true and only a sample of what I encountered in twenty years of practice. Every doctor has many to tell, and we often swap them at get-togethers — without names, of course; patient confidentiality is sacrosanct for doctors. But humour is important. We can't always take things seriously. We have to laugh at ourselves and the situations we find ourselves in. Laughter *is* the best medicine. The happiest patients I had were those who laughed easily and could find humour in life.

Of course, being happy does not mean being healthy. But humour and attitude sure helped my patients cope with illness and death.

Roy was religious and always smiling; he always had a joke and was always grateful and courteous. So it was painful to me when he developed cancer of the pancreas. He kept his smile even as his health deteriorated. He didn't need to be healthy to smile. He believed in God and was sure of his afterlife. It must have been hard to be happy, because the pain was intense and I had to start a morphine pump, a small automatic device that attaches to a person and delivers morphine at prescribed doses and times. He was constipated, nauseated, and weak. Yet Roy smiled.

One day when I came to visit, Roy was outside. His condition had deteriorated and I'd had to increase the morphine. I had expected to find Roy in bed, emaciated, half aware of his own presence. Instead I found him sitting on a stool by his fence, painting.

"It makes me happy to paint my fence," he said.

I could not stop smiling along with him as I watched him paint. He told me a story about dancing at his church and all the old ladies laughing at his antics and giving him kisses. And he continued to paint. He didn't need me that day. I would never be able to help him more than that fence did.

He died a week later. It's not easy to leave this world, but no one left it with more grace than Roy.

I think my patients taught me to laugh more, to not take life so seriously. It's easier to smile than to frown, to laugh than to cry — it's a choice. I thank all my patients for giving me more laughs than tears, more smiles than frowns, and the ability to find inner peace.

Humour and laughter were the medicines I needed when I was locked in.

CHAPTER 26
NOVEMBER TO DECEMBER: CHRISTMAS

Butterflies emerge from cocoons; I was anything but a butterfly. And I was only partially out of my shell. I feared I would never achieve my dream of walking out of the rehabilitation centre. I knew I was lucky to have gotten this far, but as humans, we always dream and want more.

A fellow who was a brainstem stroke survivor came to visit me. He had travelled quite a distance and I was most appreciative that he had gone to all that trouble. I could see he sincerely wanted to lend me support, but he walked and talked normally, and I admit I found this irritating. I discovered that he had been walking by my chronological stroke age. He was one of the few brainstem stroke survivors to regain perfectly normal function that I had read about in the medical articles at that time. I knew I would never be like him; my progress had slowed down enormously. (Since the time of my stroke, with improved clot-busting medication and acute stroke management protocol, more people are surviving a brainstem stroke with less impairment.)

Family conferences were held periodically for patients in Stan Cassidy. The whole care team — doctor, nurse, occupational therapist, and so on — met with the patient and family to discuss progress, problems, and plans. When my conference came up at the end of November, I entered it with mixed feelings. I didn't want to leave Stan Cassidy — I knew I would never get such intensive therapy as an outpatient in Saint John — yet I knew my progress was slowing and I expected to be discharged.

They wanted me to stay. They agreed my progress had slowed down, but they felt I was still progressing. I was happy they felt progress could still be made, and I wanted to stay, although I wasn't sure they were right. Probably all stroke survivors feel a sense of letdown at this phase. The quick recovery phase has ended, but that is not to say progress has finished. The recovery from this point on is painful, slow, and frustrating. It takes more effort, will, and determination, but it can happen. Besides, my physiatrist informed me that a new drug was being released for spasticity and we could try it after Christmas. This excited me; spasticity and tone were the enemy, holding me imprisoned in my own body. I didn't know what the ransom was, but I was willing to pay, whatever the price.

I extended my right arm for the first time in physiotherapy shortly after this meeting. My elbow had been bent for months. My biceps muscle was constantly contracted, making it hard for my extensors, the muscles behind my upper arm, to work. I felt as though this were a sign saying, "Don't give up. Progress can still happen."

Other things improved, such as my pivoting while holding the walker, and I could take some shirts off by myself. The act of dressing and undressing surprised me. I thought there must be some formalized set of instructions for disabled people to remove shirts independently, like the directions for making a Windsor knot in a necktie. No such luck. There are some rules, like taking the affected arm out last — or in my case, the least affected arm — but largely, it's brute strength. Pull, grab, grunt, pull again, and basically that's it. Not very scientific; just a lot of work.

I could open my mouth a little more, and the tip of my tongue could be seen when I attempted to stick it out. But spasticity of my jaw muscles made me grind my teeth so much that my canine teeth had flattened and looked like the end of a lollipop stick. Spasticity was especially bothersome in the morning. When I awoke, my whole body would contract, including my masseter muscles, responsible for chewing. I could barely open my mouth, and even my vocal cord muscles were tight, making my voice inaudible or squeaky at best.

I had better control over my emotions. Another student nurse was assigned to my care for a week, and near the end of her time with me, she, like the one before her, had to ask me questions as part of her course. This time I didn't cry — she did. I was able to talk about sex, my kids, my wife, God, and other topics without bawling. I didn't cry when I left home at the end of the weekend anymore. I could feel sad without crying or happy without laughing. It had taken six months. I didn't have control of much of my body, but at least I had control of my mind, my thoughts, and now my emotions. I felt more human.

Stan Cassidy closed for three weeks over Christmas, so I would be home for a while. It would give me a good break from the routine of institutionalized care and a chance to be with my family. I became excited as the time for Christmas break neared. I needed a change, but I was also worried about how much of a burden I would be to Jill. I was scared to find out.

Jill was more anxious than I was. She felt the stress of being totally responsible for my care and not having backup. The kids were still at school or university, so during the day she had no helpers. I knew this was a hurdle she would have to face, taking a loved one home from institutionalized care and being responsible for their total care.

I had observed this over the years in my own practice: A loved one is in hospital for many months after a life-altering illness, and finally the time comes for the patient to go home. The family then starts to make excuses why the patient can't go home, or they put up roadblocks in the way of discharge. Underneath these obstacles, the truth is that they are afraid. Once they are home and settled, things usually work out; anxieties are relieved and the patient often improves by being home.

I was very confident in Jill's ability to look after me, but I was worried that I would prove to require too much care for Jill alone and would need a full-time attendant. I really didn't think so, but the possibility was in the back of my mind.

The first day we were home, I shook Jill's confidence by falling. She was helping me up from bed after my stretching exercises when my legs gave out. I didn't hurt myself; it actually felt good to be on the floor, as silly as that sounds. Jill was very concerned and tried to help me up, but I was useless and too heavy for her to lift. It was noon and a friend of mine worked nearby. He and his wife came over and helped me up. That was the only time I fell in those three weeks. Unfortunately, it had happened on the first day, which didn't do much for Jill's confidence.

Jill did fine, as I knew she would, but I *was* a burden. We got rid of the small hospital bed and purchased a queen-sized electronic bed that enabled Jill to sleep beside me for the first time in six months. It felt so good to be back with her. I had missed her presence: the hugs, the goodnight kiss, the talks before sleep, her breathing.

I was as excited as a newlywed (well, maybe not quite that excited) to be going to bed with Jill. I loved her so and it was great, but I broke the enchantment by requesting a turn every few hours. I still required a pillow at my back or I would fall over, but I no longer needed a pillow between my knees and could sleep with my head lower. Usually, I asked the nurses at Stan Cassidy to turn me twice a night, some nights more, some less, but I had no ability to turn myself.

At home, I had to wake Jill up two or three times a night. I realized we couldn't do this forever, so when I returned to Stan Cassidy after Christmas, I asked my occupational therapist to focus on helping me learn how to turn in bed by myself. I tried to stay in one position all night, but because I couldn't shift even a little, my hips became so sore that I had to move.

I was afraid Jill was becoming tired, and I feared what effect my stroke might have on our relationship. I knew the statistics: 50 percent of marriages end in divorce after stroke. It's not hard to see why this happens: sometimes a stroke changes the survivor's personality because of where in the brain the damage occurred; sometimes the survivor's personality changes because they are mad at the world; sometimes the caregiver's personality changes because they are mad at being given a new role they didn't ask for. There are a lot of reasons why marriages break down. Jill and I had had a solid partnership up until now, and we hardly ever argued. But relationships can change.

I was incapable of turning and cuddling with Jill as we went to sleep. I was incapable of talking about the day or planning for tomorrow. I was incapable of turning over and kissing Jill goodnight. I was incapable of tenderly making love. Instead, it seemed to me, I was a burden for Jill. She had to help me into bed and position me, and then I broke her sleep by having to turn throughout the night. I hated my new role. It made me feel reduced. I was no longer the protector, the "man"; instead Jill now had to protect me.

I worried about our future, and for one night that worry turned to anger. There was nothing Jill could do to please me, and I lashed out. I wanted to be the "man." I wanted to turn and hug Jill, stroke her back, cuddle. Instead, I had to wait for a hug, for a kiss. And I had no way of showing her I wanted to make love; either I just had to say it, which sounded so cold and contrived, or Jill had to initiate the act.

Like always, Jill saw through my anger and reacted not with irritation, but with tenderness. We talked and I realized what was wrong: my role had changed and I had to accept it.

It is hard to accept these kinds of changes in your life, and I have no magic formula for my fellow stroke survivors, but we have to adapt. Love is worth the effort.

I was very happy that Christmas, despite my blow-up that one night. In fact, it was probably my happiest Christmas ever. I was thankful to be alive and to be spending another Christmas with my family. CBC Radio came to interview me, and I told them I was happy and my spirit felt light. Yes, that was how I felt: light. No burdens were weighing me down; I was giddy with happiness; I was in love with life; my spirit felt light.

I have always loved the Christmas season, but that year had special meaning for me. The carols, old and familiar as they were, seemed fresh. The Christmas lights seemed brighter and the tree scent more poignant. People seemed merrier, our parents dearer, and my children more lovable. Jill was my soulmate; it was impossible to feel closer to any other human being.

Friends visited, I went to church, and I went on outings. I visited old patients, I met old patients at malls, and I visited nursing homes I used to attend. I went to the historic Saint John City Market, where the smells and sights assaulted me. I was tormented by the food on display. I was still able to manage only puréed food, and all the fruits, baked goods, cheeses, and meats taunted me.

I tasted a beer for the first time since my stroke. I loved the taste of beer, yet I had forgotten the smell, and I spent five minutes lingering over my glass, just smelling it. The alcohol content of my first sip sent my throat into spasms, and I coughed and hacked most of it up. I took a smaller sip on my next attempt; reluctantly my throat accepted it and swallowed. But the taste! My taste buds danced. It was like the taste experience of my very first beer, only pleasant. Since that Christmas, I don't often drink beer. It's still difficult to swallow and I have to sip it. Besides, even one beer slurs my speech and makes me weak. Oh well, just another thing in my life I've had to adjust to.

Speaking of adjustments, I had to watch my family pick out a Christmas tree and then put it up and decorate it. That was painful. When they picked the tree out at a local lot, I tried not to say anything, but honestly, it was the worst-looking tree I'd ever seen. And then I had to remain quiet as I watched Jill and Colin struggle to put it up. They would probably say I didn't keep quiet, but that's not true! I used to love helping with the Christmas decorating. It was never a chore; it was festive, a family thing, and I missed partaking in that joy. Oh well, just another thing ... Adjusting! Always adjusting!

Every Christmas Eve, I've read *The Night Before Christmas* and *How the Grinch Stole Christmas* to our kids. Reading the Grinch, I would use a grinchy voice when he spoke; I didn't have to improvise this year. I didn't have the stamina to read the whole poem or story, so we took turns reading a page at a time. We laughed forever that night. Even Colin, by then a young man of twenty, took part. Young men have such a hard time showing emotions, especially with their parents. I appreciated his participation.

The kids went to bed, and it was now time for Mom and Dad to act like Santa. I only watched as Jill laid out our gifts to the children. I was feeling pretty useless, but that didn't dampen my spirits. My so-called adjustments only made me more determined to improve so I could be more helpful the next Christmas season.

It was a white Christmas. The snow had come early that year and stayed. I felt warm in spirit that Christmas morning as I watched my family opening up gifts, saying "Thank you!" and "Oh, I love this!" They had to help me open my gifts, but they seemed genuinely delighted in doing that, turning them over in my lap or holding an article of clothing up to my chest so I could see what it looked like. We smiled a lot that morning, and I was thankful to be there.

Later in the day, my parents came over for Christmas dinner. The smell of the turkey cooking all day had driven me crazy. I didn't want puréed turkey again; I wanted the whole enchilada. I knew I couldn't, so Jill compromised with me: instead of puréeing it, she diced up the turkey fine. I had mashed potatoes, squash, peas, carrots, jellied salad, dressing, and turkey. It actually looked like food. I choked a bit over the turkey but it was worth it; it was a big step for me, and I celebrated with a little wine, which I promptly choked on. I was thankful and thanked God for allowing me this time with my family.

A few days later, Jill's father and mother, her three sisters and their husbands, and our nieces and nephews from Prince Edward Island and Halifax came for a day. I had more family to celebrate with, and we laughed and joked like always. Nothing had changed, really. The only differences were that I was in a wheelchair and I couldn't talk as well, but they treated me like Shawn. They didn't patronize me or spare me as the brunt of their jokes. They seemed to feel comfortable with me, and I did with them. I was sorry when they had to head home. Their visit had brought energy, and with their absence, I was left to contemplate my return to Stan Cassidy.

I wanted to return because I wanted to improve, and now I had new goals, but still, I had to leave my family. The three weeks had flown by and the seven months before had crawled. *Seven months ago, I was happily running down those stairs on my way to work. The day was beautiful, full of promise ... Oh why? Why?* I remembered the days lying in the NICU, smothering, hot, daydream-like, unfocused. I couldn't believe that had been my experience. It seemed unreal and at the same time very much real. Thinking. Thinking. Always thinking. I wanted to be rid of those memories, but I knew I never would be. Locked in: a part of my life I never wanted to think about again, but I had no choice. It was now part of my life story.

Heading back to Stan Cassidy made me reflect on my situation. I wished I could stay home and forget about it, but I was driven to improve. I had hope, and with the introduction of new medication, my hope had foundation. *I feel I'm going to walk. I will.*

CHAPTER 27
JANUARY TO MARCH: FRUSTRATIONS AND MUSIC

On my return to Stan Cassidy, Todd and I again shared a room. This pleased me; I found him to be a very pleasant young man, and we shared many a laugh.

I quickly returned to the routine: the wake-up call, the therapy schedule board, the meals, the long evenings, and finally the bedtime routine. The white-cement walls felt colder, the bathrooms smaller, and the cafeteria more sterile. However, the staff still glowed with warmth, and it was not long before Denis had me laughing and Louise had me smiling and I shook off my melancholy mood.

The nursing staff was special; each person brought something from their own personality that helped me. I could write about each one and the unique gifts they brought to work every day. They became almost maternal (or paternal) as they taught me how to wash my face, shave, brush my teeth, and do all the personal tasks my own mother had once taught me. Some were better than others at teaching. Some brought humour; some did not. Some shared stories of their families; some were private.

Some were happy in their own lives; some were not. But they all brought kindness and compassion and smiles.

I still had my "main girls," Beth, Mereille, and Doreen, and they were happy to see I hadn't lost any function in the three weeks I was home. My daughters, Beth and Tara, had done my stretching exercises most days, giving Jill a break. I was proud and touched to have my daughters perform physiotherapy on my limbs. They were not timid in touching their dad like I had thought they might be. Rather, they pulled, lifted, twisted, and pushed my limbs with great gusto.

I entered my therapies with a renewed sense of determination. I could tell my speech was slowly improving, and I wanted to work harder on my breath support and pronunciation. I had two main goals I wanted physiotherapy and occupational therapy to help me with: I wanted to be able to turn in bed by myself and to be independent moving my wheelchair. I also wanted to walk, but I kept this secret to myself. I thought it might be possible if the new medication reduced my tone, but I didn't want to verbalize my hopes. It's harder to act nonchalant in failure if everyone knows your goal.

It wasn't hard to keep a secret; no one understood what I was saying, anyway. I was introduced to Tracy, a speech language pathologist I had not yet met. Apparently, Beth had been covering for Tracy during her pregnancy leave. I still saw Beth once a week, but I worked with Tracy daily. Tracy was a young woman whose pleasant nature didn't soften her approach; she was every bit as hard a taskmaster as Beth.

After weeks of individual sessions, Tracy decided to try me in a group. I still saw Beth weekly for private work, but I went to group twice a week. Most of the exercises that the speech therapists gave me to increase my breath support were difficult to do daily and stay motivated. The improvements didn't occur every week, barely every month, and it was hard to repeat exercises with no positive reward or visual gains. This was not unique to speech therapy; all rehabilitation was like this, to some degree. I had to keep reminding myself that at the very least I was strengthening any functions I'd gained.

I was still stubbornly against buying a power chair. Over Christmas I'd tried to manoeuvre independently in my home, but after a length of time — measured by my tolerance for frustration — I would call Jill or one of the kids for help. Had I tried long enough? If they hadn't been there, would I have succeeded, or would I still be stuck in the same place? These types of questions made me reluctant to order a power wheelchair.

I was no further ahead with my ability to walk. Jill, Betty, Doreen, and Mereille continued to be my entourage as I "walked" through the gym. They stayed positive and Mereille observed small improvements, but I saw little to be joyful about. I did start to swing my back leg up to meet my front leg, but that was occasional and took a lot of effort. My legs refused to relax and bend. Unless they loosened up a bit, I would never walk.

I eagerly awaited the introduction of this new medicine to my drug schedule. Perhaps it would be my ticket to freedom.

Tizanidine was the new antispasmodic drug that I was hoping would reduce my tone better than the one I was currently taking and jump-start my rehabilitation. It had just been approved for use in Canada. It has a nasty side effect of drowsiness, so it has to be started slowly, and then the dosage can be increased incrementally until the desired effect or the maximum dose is reached. Some people are not bothered by drowsiness or other side effects, some people's bodies accommodate to the side effects, and some people never adapt to the drug.

The idiosyncratic nature of drug behaviour in the human body was always apparent to me when treating hypertension, or high blood pressure. Treating hypertension can be life saving, and at the very least, lowering blood pressure reduces a risk factor for many diseases. However, hypertension as a disease usually has no symptoms, and it is difficult giving a drug to patients who feel well, subjecting them to potential side effects. The goal always is to find a drug that causes no side effects for that individual. The physician and the patient have to work together to reach that goal of treating hypertension effectively while minimizing the side effects. And sometimes, some side effects have to be accepted for the greater benefit.

My physiatrist started me on a low dose of tizanidine, as recommended. For the first few days, I was drowsy. I had expected this, but in the past my body had quickly adapted to drugs, so I wasn't alarmed. Although I was still drowsy after a few days, I implored the physiatrist to increase the dose anyway. The drowsiness increased. I could barely keep my eyes open as Betty and Esmond stretched my limbs after breakfast. I often fell asleep for short periods and then awoke as they reached my pain threshold for the stretched limb.

My voice, which had been improving, became slurred and unintelligible until the drug wore off. And tizanidine was not reducing my tone enough to improve my function.

I held on for three weeks. I was determined to make it work. I had such great hope for recovery by using tizanidine, but now those hopes were being tested.

Don't get me wrong: I wasn't expecting that tizanidine would cure me. I knew it would not take the place of hard work, but I had hoped it would reduce the tone more and thereby enable me to work my spastic limbs better. If anything, the drowsiness and tiredness were worsening, not improving, with time, so reluctantly I asked the physiatrist to take me off it.

I did not realize what a fog I had been in for the three weeks I was on tizanidine until I came off it. It's a very good drug for some people and has made a tremendous difference in their lives. My experience was not great, but I would have no hesitation recommending it to a patient. I would caution them about potential side effects, but that would not prevent me from trying it.

My physiatrist decided to increase the dosage of my initial antispasmodic, baclofen, so I still had hope that my tone could be reduced — or at least that the spasticity would lessen over time. Baclofen made me drowsy, too, but not to the extent tizanidine did. Slowly, we eventually reached the recommended maximum dose and beyond, but sadly it never significantly reduced the tone in my muscles for functional gain.

However, I did not give up on tizanidine completely. I tried it five more times over the year, and each time the results were the same: it was a battle to remain awake. I wanted so much for something to work, to reduce my tone so I could improve. After the fifth attempt, I had to accept that the drug and I didn't mix. I have tried weight-bearing exercises to reduce tone, and medication delivered directly to my spine, all with limited success. I've learned not to set my hopes as high with new treatments as I did with tizanidine.

Another drug that concerned me was zopiclone, the sleeping medication I started using early on in my illness. As I've said, my sleeping mechanism went awry with my stroke, and it took a while to find a sleeping pill that worked.

My physiatrist assured me that my insomnia would get better with time. I have seen patients become dependent on sleeping pills and then develop tolerance to them, needing more or stronger medication for the same effect, and so a struggle ensues. Sleeping medication should be prescribed for short-term use only. I was determined I would not become dependent.

In the fall, I had started to cut down my zopiclone to half the dosage. After my body had accommodated to that reduction and I was still sleeping, I stopped taking it. My body had repaired itself; I slept well and wasn't dependent on medication.

I walked poorly during the first part of February with Mereille. Doreen concentrated on my sit-to-stand ability, but I failed. My back would still not let me bend enough to keep my weight forward to move from sitting to standing. I still experienced the same problem: when I put effort into using my legs to stand, my back extended, throwing my weight backward. My brain knew what had to be done, but my body didn't listen. No matter how hard I told myself to keep my hips bent and my chest forward, my back would extend. I had no control, and the harder I tried, the worse I did.

Doreen knew I would gain a lot of independence by being able to stand up on my own. And I was so close. I could stand without help from a certain height, but not from the level of a bed or wheelchair. Twenty years later, I cannot stand independently from these levels unless I'm holding on to something, and even then, it's sometimes risky.

I had stood by myself, holding on to a bar, for the first time in December, and as with most accomplishments in stroke, I thought this was only the beginning. I thought if I kept working at sit-to-stand, I would progress. Sad to say, it doesn't always work out that way. It was the same old story: I got discouraged because I wasn't improving, but I couldn't give up. If I were to succumb to frustration and stop trying, I would certainly fail.

I couldn't flex my hips to bring my knees up to turn in bed. Mereille would bend my hips when I failed and then I tried rocking my knees back and forth to turn. Sometimes with great effort I did turn over, only to have my legs and back now sticking out straight in extension and my right arm tightly curled up in spasmodic protest. From this position, Mereille wanted me to kick my legs over the bed, put my arm under my body and lift myself up into sitting position. The best I could do was smile sweetly at her.

I still didn't have 100 percent control over my bladder. I didn't wear adult diapers anymore, but I had urgency — when I had to go, I had to go. One night, I awoke needing to urinate but couldn't find the call bell, and before I could awaken Todd to ring for help, I let go. Because there was no sense in waking Todd now, I lay in the wet bed for a few hours, until some nurses came in to attend to my friend. I had thought I had good urinary control, but this belief was shaken by this incident and then once at home and on another evening at Stan Cassidy. Two steps forward, one step back. Two steps forward, one step back. Always. Frustrating.

I tried to be independent. One morning after breakfast, I went into the bathroom by myself, in my power chair, brushed my teeth, cleaned up a bit, urinated using the urinal, congratulated myself, and headed out. A nurse had closed the bathroom door after she had come in for some towels while I was brushing my teeth, and now I was stuck. I couldn't bend forward enough to grab the door handle, and the room was too small to turn sideways to the door. The emergency bell was located behind the toilet and I couldn't reach the cord. My voice wasn't loud enough to be heard, so I kept banging into the door with my power chair, hoping someone would hear me. Half an hour later, someone did hear and came to my rescue.

This happened twice.

So, as you can see, by early February, I was frustrated and disappointed. Disappointed because I couldn't take tizanidine; frustrated by my lack of progress and the events that had transpired.

I didn't entertain the thought of giving up, though. I hoped this was just a lull in my progress, but I admit, I was discouraged.

Mereille's and Doreen's attitudes were especially important to me during this time. Their humour and positivity sustained me.

My discharge date was coming up — February 11 — and I was ready to go. After all, I had come back to try the tizanidine. The trial had failed, so I thought I was due to go. My physiatrist came to watch me walk, and after consulting with Mereille, he concluded he wanted me to stay until the end of March. They had seen some improvements recently and wanted to work on them. Apparently, they saw improvements in my walking! I didn't see it, but I was more than willing to stay if there was a chance of walking.

Besides, not everything was negative. I moved my right arm up to touch my face for the first time and my left arm was stronger. My balance was terrible, but my legs were getting stronger. I could turn pages better, lift a cup to my mouth, wash, shave — all better. My emotions were fully under control now, and I could listen to music again.

Music has always been an important part of my life. I started playing guitar in grade nine when I asked for an electric guitar and amplifier from the Sears catalogue for Christmas. It had two pickups and a sunburst finish. The amplifier had a whopping five watts, but that proved to be more than loud enough, according to my parents. The action — the ease of pressing a string to a fret — was horrible, but I was in heaven.

My musical tastes gradually changed from electric to acoustic over the years. I was self-taught, never very good. I didn't try to be good — I played for my enjoyment only and I sounded good enough for me. In high school I liked the Beatles, Rolling Stones, and later Led Zeppelin. In my university days I started playing more Cat Stevens, Paul Simon, and Neil Young. I strummed or fingerpicked the guitar and sang. I never could sing well, but my family will tell you it wasn't from lack of trying. I loved playing my guitar and singing. It was what I did to relax.

We bought a piano because Jill plays and we wanted our children to learn. I learned to adapt my knowledge of guitar chords to the piano. I played them with my right hand while doing a bass run with my left and singing the melody. I had great fun doing this, too, although my kids preferred me to play guitar — at least I was in my room, by myself! But the guitar was my love.

It was almost a compulsion. I had to feel the guitar neck in my hand at least once a day. I had to pick the darn thing up, even if only for five minutes. I remember working in the office all day, going to the ER for an evening shift, coming home tired at midnight, and still picking it up to play something quiet while I unwound.

Jill said she could always tell what mood I was in by what I played. If I came home angry or disturbed about something that had occurred, an angry Neil Young song would come out. If I was melancholy, it was bluesy or a quiet Neil Young or Bob Dylan or Paul Simon song. If I was happy, she'd hear "The 59th Street Bridge Song (Feelin' Groovy)" by Simon and Garfunkel or "Cinnamon Girl" by Neil Young. I sometimes became studious and played a Beatles melody in classical style or attempted a Michael Hedges or Leo Kottke tune. I enjoyed writing my own songs — never serious, never recorded, often forgotten after a few days, but fun and probably cathartic.

When I was a young man, I vowed I would buy a Martin guitar when I could afford it. And I did. I loved my Martin guitar; I loved the look, sound, feel, even the smell of it. When I had my stroke, it felt strange not to have my guitar nearby, but it didn't bother me as much as I would have thought. I was unable to play and I accepted this, or at least I thought I did.

I thought one of the good things about coming home on the weekends, that first summer, would be the ability to play my own music. At Stan Cassidy, I gave up playing CDs in the portable player because I often ended up with the headphones on my head for a considerable amount of time after the CD was finished. I imagined myself lying back in my own room, listening to my CDs, while I waited for my tube feedings to be finished. No headphones to contend with, and I could listen without disturbing anyone.

Jill put on a Blue Rodeo CD and I settled back for an enjoyable, relaxing few moments — then I started to cry. A familiar guitar part rang out, one that I had learned and played many times. It brought back too many memories, too many emotions, all in an instant, and I wasn't ready. My tears were unexpected. I had thought I had this guitar absence under control. I had to ring my bell for Jill to return and turn off the CD. Over the weeks, I tried other CDs and genres of music, but the results were always the same.

At Stan Cassidy, Louise thought I didn't like country music (not that I didn't like it; I had never been exposed to it), so as a joke she often played country music while she helped me prepare for the day. I groaned, pretending to be annoyed, but in actuality, I didn't mind it at all. Country music brought back no memories for me, and it became the bridge to tunes I used to listen to.

I bought a narrow-bodied guitar and tried playing it in the hope that would awaken memories between my brain and fingers, but it failed. My right arm refused to move from its flexed, contracted position to strum, and my fingers refused to move to pick the strings. I tried this because I saw my father-in-law regain his ability to play the piano after a stroke. He was a good piano player, and the inability to play piano was quite devastating for him. I saw him practise and practise, over and over, until he got that right hand back to almost normal function. At first, I didn't think he would do it. I was afraid he was frustrating himself with an unobtainable goal. But he did it.

There seems to be intangibles involved when we are discussing the mind and music. My soul seems to want music. I heard classical music that first day after I awoke from my coma. Did my mind invent it? Or did I *hear* it? While I lay in the NICU, I intuitively wanted to listen to nature CDs, even though I've never listened to them before. My soul seemed to want the tranquility.

Music is fascinating: the many varieties, the tones, the way it makes you feel. Music, like love, is food for the soul, and my soul seems to be in a feeding frenzy lately. Classical, jazz, pop, rock — anything goes and everything feels right.

CHAPTER 28
JANUARY TO MARCH:
LOVE

At home I requested to be moved to our sofa or a chair less frequently. I was growing comfortable being in the wheelchair. I no longer felt trapped, confined. This acceptance was a slow process and I wasn't aware of any stages, but I prefer being in my chair now — I find it more comfortable than a normal chair. Now I have to remind myself that I can sit on a different chair occasionally. I once thought I would never get used to a wheelchair. I guess if there is no option, the body can adapt to almost anything.

I had no more falls at home, and Jill became confident in her ability to look after me. I did sort of fall one more time, one evening when we were practising walking. My pants were wedged, and I asked Jill to pull them down. As a joke, she pulled my pants and underwear down in one quick swoop. I became weak with laughter and slowly buckled to the floor. Jill tried to keep me up but was laughing too hard herself. I ended up sitting on the floor with a bare bottom. After I wrapped myself with a towel, Beth and Tara helped Jill to get me up. We had some explaining to do!

We try not to be too jovial while I'm on my feet. Laughter literally makes my knees go weak.

I watched very little television. I guess I overdosed on those electron images while I was locked in. I exercised, read, or spent time on the computer, where I discovered a site on the internet for stroke survivors to interact, and specifically a place for brainstem stroke survivors. I found many people like me across North America. Many of the brainstem stroke survivors were young. The common bonds of experiences, fears, and hopes linked us together.

I connected with Jim's wife. Jim was the man I had read about who stopped his tube feedings. His wife started to correspond with me in September, and by January it became apparent to me that he wasn't responding; he continued to be locked in. I found it hard to say anything. It was tough to be encouraging, because I knew his hopes of recovery were fading, yet that was what she was asking for. I didn't want to give her the cold facts because they were cruel, but I've seen well-meaning people be too hopeful: "He'll get better," "Have faith," "Tell him to fight." I tried to be supportive for her without resorting to clichés, but I wanted to say, *Maybe he won't get better. It's not his fault if he doesn't improve. Sometimes there's nothing to fight with.* I didn't want her to lose hope, but she had to be told his chances for some recovery were dimming as time marched on.

Jim could communicate with the eye-gaze board like I had, and by June, he'd made the decision to end his life. He had not improved. He was still quite locked in and declared he didn't want to live. He asked to stop his tube feeds, except for water, and he quietly passed away a few weeks later. Thankfully, no one made a fuss about this being amoral, and he was allowed to carry out his wishes.

I don't know about the morality of assisted suicide anymore. Would it have been more humane to assist him in dying by suicide quickly, instead of lingering for a few weeks? Undoubtedly, it would have been more humane, but would it have been moral? Until society or theologians can work this out, we are safer in accepting this form of passive suicide. Since I first wrote these words, the Government of Canada has made medical assistance in dying legal under certain situations, and many deaths have taken place under this new law. I am in favour of this and would like to see medical assistance in dying extended to provide for advance directives. However, the new laws wouldn't have helped me in my circumstance, as I had no prognosis of inevitable, foreseeable death.

I could not help but ask myself whether I would have done the same thing as Jim if I had stayed locked in. I think I would have. I don't think I could have lived only being able to move my eyes, never smiling, unable to kiss, unable to hug. I think those who live this way must be very courageous, perhaps strong in their faith. I don't know if suicide is amoral; I think I would have taken my chances. If God is forgiving, perhaps he would understand my reasons for taking my own life. That it was hell living locked in. Yes, I would have taken my chances.

I think back to that Saturday in the summer: if I'd had a way, would I have taken my life that day? I don't think so, but my soul was pretty black. That would have been wrong, and that is why impulsive suicide has to be prevented. A person who is depressed and suicidal may think differently after they've been successfully treated. But that is different from a person who suffers from a terminal or hopeless situation contemplating suicide. Surely we've progressed enough in our judgments to be able to distinguish between the two circumstances.

Stroke survivors post their stories on the stroke website, and often people will privately ask us for our advice. The danger of the internet is that people may pose as someone they're not. I can tell that people on the site often aren't sure whether to believe I am really a doctor.

One question I often get asked is "How did you get through it?" I'm sure I've disappointed people with my response. I tried to think of some clever medical-psychological answer, but I never found one. When I've been pressured to respond, my reply is quite simple, perhaps clichéd or corny, but it was my honest answer — the same damn thing you've heard time after time, in song after song, in sermon after sermon, in whisper after whisper: love.

I hear John Lennon singing that love is the answer.

Love — so hard to find, so confusing, and so very important in our lives, as I found out. I envy those who find love that lasts forever with their first sweetheart. Before I met Jill, there was one girl I was sure was *the one*. I was astonished to find out I was wrong, and even more astonished to find out I was to blame for the breakup.

Shortly after my high-school sweetheart and I broke up after three years together, I met a new girl at university. We had a two-year relationship that ended suddenly, and I never figured out why. But after I came out of my coma and while I was locked in, the answer to the great mystery of my life became clear to me. I don't know if I was visited by spirits and shown my transgressions like Scrooge was, or if another spiritual thing happened, or if I just had time to think and revisit my past. The answer was so crystal clear: I didn't call her once that whole summer while I was home working. Duh!

I must have thought that once I'd found love, it stood on its own. Wrong! Love has to be watered to be sustained and grow, or it will wither. I had four significant relationships before I met

Jill, and now I can see I was guilty of not sharing myself totally in any of them.

My first love I took for granted, assuming she'd always be there. I didn't put enough effort into showing her how much I loved her. With my second love, I subconsciously tested our bond repeatedly. To my third love I gave nothing of myself, unconsciously preparing for the inevitable breakup. And with my fourth love, I looked for and imagined signs of impending breakup and initiated the dissolution myself.

I loved all these girls; they were wonderful people, and I have to take most of the blame for abusing or ignoring love. I never showed any of them the whole me. I didn't understand my phobias, anxieties, and panic attacks, and I was in denial about them. I was embarrassed and hid the total me. I think my girlfriends felt this, that there was something missing. For love to flourish, I had to be vulnerable, show them the whole me, warts and all, fears and dreams.

Perhaps the six-year-old Shawn inside me was still so paranoid about parental loss that he hung back from relationships, unable to give anyone control over his well-being again, suspicious of truly lasting love. I also didn't take time to mourn my failed relationships. Maybe young Shawn was avoiding potential flashbacks to parental loss by dating a new girl within weeks of the last one. This was an amazing feat, considering I'm nothing to look at, which, combined with my low self-esteem, made the task of asking a girl out on a date an angst-ridden, difficult job for me. Was my subconscious desperation to avoid dealing with relationship loss so great that I could overcome the anxiety of asking a girl out?

After my fourth significant relationship ended — they were getting shorter in length as time went on, from nearly four years for the first one to four months for the last — I wisely avoided girls for nearly two years.

Perhaps it was all karma; I was to find my forever soulmate in Jill.

I saw Jill in my first days in medical school. My medical class got together one evening for a social event to get to know each other. Before the social, we assembled in our large lecture theatre to hear a few students from second year give us their perspective on first year and what textbooks to buy. Their girlfriends or boyfriends came with them, to attend the social event immediately after.

They all seemed quite confident — after all, they had made it through the first year — but there was one girl who didn't seem as confident as the rest. She was pretty, with dark-blond hair, and was wearing a white top with blue jeans and sneakers. She seemed as if she'd be a pleasant, kind soul.

There were many other people there but I remembered only her. She seemed uncomfortable standing in front of about a hundred medical students. I understood her discomfort; I would have felt the same. She was the girlfriend of one of the second-year fellows, but he seemed so confident and she seemed so unlike him. I liked her, whoever she was.

I was looking at my future wife, Jill.

She doesn't remember any of it. Darn! I thought she might have spotted me in the crowd of medical students and was enchanted right there — a perfect fairy tale.

I did not see this girl again for more than a year. At a party one night, one of my classmates introduced me to a friend of hers. I recognized her immediately — it was Jill. I knew that I would like her, and I did. I immediately found her easy to talk to; I felt comfortable in her presence.

Apparently she had broken up with her boyfriend, but I wasn't sure. We stayed as friends for more than a year. Jill worked as a nurse at the Izaak Walton Killam Hospital for Children, and

I often saw and spoke to her there. And I would see her at parties. We always talked, but I never thought of Jill in any way other than as a friend.

One time, after unexpectedly running into her and chatting, I felt the desire to get to know her better, so a few days later, I phoned to ask her out. I guess after two years I was willing to risk a broken heart. She agreed, and we went out with her roommate and her roommate's boyfriend and had a wonderful time. She was kind, but I had known that from the moment I saw her years before.

I was happy — really happy for the first time in years. Jill and I continued seeing each other, and before I went into internship, we married. We have been married forty years as I'm rewriting this memoir, and my love for her is still growing. Hopefully, I've learned something along the way; hopefully, I've remembered to water our love.

I have spent this much time talking about love because love was so important in my recovery. Jill's love for me brought me through. When I was in despair, depressed, and somewhat suicidal, it was love that brought me up from those depths. Jill didn't have to say much — her touches and smile filled my spirit.

In those early days, as I lay in the NICU, her arrival at my bedside filled me with a deep joy. It felt like the joy I had experienced the first night I went out with her, only deeper. Just looking at her makes me smile.

Jill has made me believe that any disability I might end up with was inconsequential. Love was my goal in life and I have achieved it. Everything has been secondary to the love Jill and I share.

I once said to Jill, before I had my stroke, "Know this: if I ever die suddenly, I die happy." I meant it, but at the time I had no idea how love would be the catalyst for me to work as hard as I could to rehabilitate.

And so, my simple, perhaps feeble-sounding answer to the lady who asked me "How did you get through it?" is this: love.

CHAPTER 29
JANUARY TO MARCH:
THE SPIRITUAL

Love was the basis of my acceptance and my determination to improve. It gave rise to such statements as *I don't know if I will succeed, but I do know I won't succeed if I stop trying* and *Any movement I gain, however small, is a bonus.* Love was the safety net that caught me when I failed. What more in this world could I ask for but love?

There are many different types of love that are just as important as the love Jill and I share: love between child and parent, between siblings, between friends, or for God. Love for God was important in my recovery.

I went to church as a child. My grandmother made sure I attended Sunday school at St. Luke's Anglican Church in Saint John. Reverend Quinn impressed me, with his white hair and beard and magnificent robes — white-and-black robes complemented by adornments of brilliant red or purple or other colours, depending upon the Christian season. People listened to him, and the power and sight of him made quite an impression on this quiet, scrawny kid. Becoming an Anglican priest appealed to me. People would have to listen, and I, too, could wear those fine robes. Such status was a temptation to a shy boy.

Religion took a back seat in my adolescent years. Like most teenagers, I was more concerned with the present and the immediate future. It's hard to think of abstract ideas when you are more concerned with questions such as *Who am I? What am I doing? What am I going to do in life?*

Science had more answers than religion — at least, I thought so — and I thought less and less about God. I didn't discount that there could be a God, but I thought it was improvable and I was into the scientific method. I wanted proof; faith was not enough.

In my twenties and early thirties, I was agnostic, if not an atheist at times, but really I didn't give it much thought. Also, I would have been too anxious to enter a church back then, because of my phobia over loss of control and crowds.

Jill took the kids to Saint David's United Church in Rothesay, and it was here that I started to listen to the Christian message again. The minister preached about peace, love, forgiveness, and helping others. He didn't dwell on sins, damnation, or religious doctrine and beliefs I had a hard time accepting. He reflected that how you conducted yourself, how you showed others peace, love, and forgiveness, was more important than what you believed.

This was what I needed. I couldn't blindly accept religious beliefs and dogma on faith alone; my brain wasn't wired that way. I experienced an intangible feeling that had been missing in my adult life: a familiar sense of peace I'd had as a child attending the Anglican church. At the very least, by going to church I was spending some time each week reflecting on life and thinking of people less fortunate than I was. I soon grew to love the other members of that church, and later, Jill and I taught Sunday school, dwelling mostly on the themes of love, peace, happiness, and respecting others and the moral lessons of some of the Biblical stories. I remained skeptical of many of the Biblical stories and much religious dogma, but I had an inner feeling that there was something to this God, and soon I had confirmation.

About a year before the stroke, I started to experience weird sensations. They happened about six times. I would suddenly get a feeling that something drastic was about to happen to my family. I didn't know it was a stroke, or even that the change would occur to me, but each time, I turned to Jill and said, "Something is going to happen to one of us. I just want you to know I love you, and if I die, I die happy. I've done everything I've wanted to do. We have wonderful kids and I love you."

The sensations were so clear, so definite: something was going to happen to our family.

One time this sensation came over me as I walked onto the deck at the side of our house. I turned to Jill and told her what had just happened and how I loved her. Another time it happened as I was falling asleep. I don't remember the other times specifically, because once they were over, I soon forgot about them. I did not dwell on the feelings; I was not spooked by them. I didn't even necessarily believe them. It was just one of those freaky things that happen.

I remembered the premonitions soon after I awoke from my coma. *Holy cow!* I thought. *Those feelings were true. I believe God warned me. He was preparing me. There* is *a God and he's watching us and cares for us.* This knowledge made me happy as I lay in the NICU. I don't know if it was God who told me, or loved ones in a spirit world or what, but something happened.

I feel confident in my soul that I am right; the feeling was so clear. I'd never experienced anything comparable to it before. If I am right, God is omnipresent, or perhaps there is another dimension of souls among us with limited ability to communicate. I'll go with God as the mystery, a name our ancestors used to convey that Holy Spirit.

Jill asks me, "If he's so omnipresent, why do atrocities occur, children starve or cancer exist — why? If he knew a stroke was about to happen to you, why didn't he stop it?"

I don't know the answer to these questions. Maybe he can't change events, but only our spirits. I don't know, but I do have hope that God or a spirit world exists.

When things are going well, we are often skeptical about our good fortune and comment that something bad is going to happen. We know what life is like, and we're right: nothing lasts forever in this world, and bad things happen all the time. But my experience wasn't cerebral, just a thought — it was a knowing, a revelation.

Skeptics will say I had a near-death experience, so I have embraced a fable to comfort myself. Knowing that God or something exists does give me comfort, but I had great hope in the existence of God before my stroke. I didn't need this experience to give me hope. It solidified my hope in God, it changed my thoughts on how God operates, but I didn't seize the concept of God in an act of desperation.

Some people call my experiences premonitions. What is a premonition? *Collier's Dictionary* defines the word as "an actual warning of something yet to occur," but says nothing about what this phenomenon is. Where does it come from? Do we have another sense? Is there a foreseeable pattern to our lives?

I don't think science will ever be able to explain premonition. Perhaps it is God talking to us. We are told by pastors, ministers, and priests that he talks to us more than we realize. We don't listen, or maybe we don't know how to.

Intuition. Deepak Chopra believes that listening to our intuition, our real intuition, is a stage in knowing God.

Regardless of what you believe about my spiritual experience — *Hogwash! He's a nice guy but a little flaky* — my religion did afford me comfort in my illness. I often recited Psalm 23 in those first days as I lay on the verge of death: "Even though I walk through the valley of the shadow of death ..." It gave me great comfort. I did not fear death. I was not afraid.

I wonder if everyone acts a little selfish when they are near death. I wasn't worried about Jill and my children; I was not worried about anything. And all the while, that curious music played in my head and I was at peace.

Over the successive days, weeks, and then months, I prayed every night. I asked God for strength. I resisted the temptation to ask him for a complete return to normal, not while children were dying and people were struggling for food, with addictions, with loss, with all the miseries in this world. I simply prayed for the strength to continue to work hard and not give up.

I tend to wonder about coincidences now.

CHAPTER 30
ART AND HILDA

Art and Hilda — I inherited them from another physician who had left town. By this time, Art had already suffered two strokes. He walked with a quad cane, which has a platform with four rubber ends for greater stability, and his affected arm was in a permanent flexed position. He spoke out of the side of his mouth.

Art loved to talk so much, I hardly got a word in during my home visits. He loved to watch the parliamentary channel on TV and then ranted on and on about what the politicians were doing wrong. The longer I let him speak, the more agitated he became and the worse his blood pressure reading would be. I learned to take his blood pressure first thing on my visits. It would invariably be much better than if I waited until after his discourse on politics.

I loved the guy; he was humorous and loved to tell me about the old days. Hilda would chide Art, telling him he had said enough and that he had to let the doctor do his work. Sometimes it was hard to get everything done, but I didn't mind. I loved to hear him talk.

Hilda was always just as friendly. She was a thinly built woman with a permanent smile. She hung on Art's every word, admonishing him for repeating a story he'd told me the month before. I could tell she worshipped him and they had had a life-long partnership of love. Their son and his family lived in the flat above them, so they had plenty of help if needed. I had a feeling Hilda didn't ask for help very often.

As the years went by, Art suffered repeated small strokes that left him more physically challenged and, sadly, more con-fused. The post-stroke dementia developed slowly. I could see his responses to my questions becoming more bizarre, and finally there was no spoken interaction. It pained me to see this once friendly, talkative, proud man become a fellow who just stared.

Hilda continued to talk to him, comb his hair, and fix his shirt so he looked presentable. The love between the two had not changed. Art was unable to show Hilda the love he felt for her, but this had not changed anything: she knew her Art was still there. Hilda was not a big woman, but still she dressed him and helped him to his favourite chair. This must have taken a lot of effort, and we had to face the facts: maybe it was time to start thinking of nursing homes, I would tell her. She would laugh gently and tell me they were doing just fine. Why, they were still going for drives!

Art had spent his life around cars and had owned a repair garage. He got visibly excited when he was going for a car ride. I couldn't imagine how she managed to get Art — now unable to walk without a lot of support — into a car.

Where did they go? Hilda told me they always went up the river road to the town of Grand Bay. There they would sit in the car and have an ice cream while watching the boats sailing on the bay. I pictured them in happier times, laughing, talking, being together. They were still in each other's company, but Hilda carried on the conversation or sometimes they sat in silence, happy just being together.

One day, Hilda showed up at my office looking rather pale, saying that she was tired. She looked ill, and I quickly arranged for some blood tests to be done. When the tests came back, they pointed to a form of leukemia. I arranged for her to be admitted to the hospital the next day. Meanwhile, Art's family upstairs would look after him.

In hospital, we found that Hilda had an especially aggressive form of leukemia. Her prognosis was poor, considering her age, but the hematologist offered her a chance with some chemotherapy. The chemo would be rough on her; would she be able to physically withstand the side effects?

I probably should have advised her not to try, but this happened so fast that I hadn't got used to the idea of Hilda being sick. I had to try something. I would have abided by her wishes, but she kept saying, "Whatever you think, doctor."

The ball was in my court and I had to go for it. "The chemo will probably make you very sick, Hilda, but it is the only chance. The hematologist wants to start tomorrow, but before he does so, he wants you to receive some blood. Your blood is very low and we need to get that up before the chemo starts. We're going to start the blood this evening and it will be finished by early morning. Okay?"

She smiled and said, "Whatever you think, doctor." She had become so frail so fast. She looked child-like, dwarfed by the pillows as she smiled sweetly at me and said goodbye.

The next morning, I was making my rounds early and I couldn't find Hilda's chart.

"Hilda died during the night," said a nurse when I asked about it. "She seemed fine at three a.m., breathing and sleeping just as good as you or me. Then when we went back about an

247

hour later, she was dead. We didn't want to bother you, so we called the doctor on call."

I always wanted them to call me if one of my patients died. At least the dreaded call to the family informing them of their loved one's passing would be from someone they knew, instead of from a total stranger. Or worse still, I feared entering the hospital to make rounds, meeting a family member, telling them I was just about to go up and see their loved one, only to hear them say, "Oh, don't you know? He died!"

I was too shocked to admonish the nurses for not calling me. I had not expected Hilda to die that night — maybe the next week, but not the night before. There had been no signs of distress or impending death when I had left. I had to make that dreaded phone call; the nurse had already called Hilda's family, but I wanted to offer any help I could and express my sympathy.

I said to her son, "Don, sorry about your mother. I didn't expect it or I would have called you last evening. Probably for the best. She would have suffered with the chemo. Apparently she passed away peacefully in her sleep."

"Doc, Dad died, too."

"What! When?"

"Last night. We called the doctor who was on call for you and he came over and pronounced him dead. He had stopped eating since Mom went into hospital. He was getting weaker, but he seemed fine when we put him to bed. He died around midnight."

I suspect Hilda and Art are still having their ice cream on the hill overlooking the bay. Coincidence or not?

CHAPTER 31
JANUARY TO MARCH: HOME

Love acted as a buoy, preventing me from sinking into despair, but it didn't prevent me from feeling hopelessness. I acknowledged that the drug experiment had failed and that I was a prisoner of my muscle tone. My muscles seemed willing to relearn, but rigidity held them back.

Todd, my roommate, was discharged in early March. Underneath his youthful bravado there was a very kind and gentle soul. I was going to miss him. He left quietly without fanfare while I ate my lunch in the cafeteria. It was typical of Todd: accepting fate with little fuss. He wouldn't have wanted to be the centre of attention.

My discharge date — the end of March — held firm. I was eager to start my new life at home. Each attempt at walking became a disappointment for me. Each failed attempt at sitting or standing only emphasized the point that it was time to go home. I would receive physical therapy at the Saint John Regional Hospital as an outpatient, and I thought it was more likely that I'd make gains attempting the functional activities of daily living at home.

I had daydreamed of walking out of Stan Cassidy on my discharge date. I'd imagined that I would independently walk from my room with a walker, my legs dancing with muscle spasms, down the corridor, and stop at the front desk. There I'd wait, joking with the receptionist about her upcoming wedding while Jill brought the car to the front door. The receptionist would remark on how good it was to see me walk. I'd thank her for saying so. Jill would arrive and I'd walk out the front door and slide into the car.

It wasn't going to happen.

My secret dream of walking out of Stan Cassidy was not going to be fulfilled. It hurt, but I'd had months to reconcile myself to reality. As I said earlier, when you hit a wall, back up and go around. It was my time to try another avenue.

I decided to accept my failure for now, but that didn't mean I would never walk. *I will keep trying. I might.* I was back to the possibilities.

I wrote a short thank-you note to each nurse, nursing assistant, doctor, and therapist. I had spent nearly a year of my life in Stan Cassidy, and I owed them so much. I had taken from each a part of their personality they had to offer. From some I took their humour, others their smile, advice, sincerity, or kindness. They had helped me remain focused on life.

I thought back to those dark, ugly days of being locked in, brightened by the staff with smiles, jokes, and hugs. I had so much to be grateful for. I had come through a tunnel so narrow that my thoughts had seemed imprisoned. Every health professional and supportive staff member had been instrumental in pulling me through.

I had become dependent upon my therapists, especially Mereille. I came to think of her as my angel, a light to help me through those difficult times. And perhaps that is what angels are:

people we don't expect coming forward and guiding us through difficult times.

Mereille cried when I said farewell and thanked her for all she'd done. I didn't cry. I'm not saying that was a good thing, but it meant I was finally in command of my emotions. I easily broke away from Mereille, Doreen, Beth, Tracy, my physiatrist, and all the nursing staff.

It felt odd to look back at Stan Cassidy as we drove away. The little white-cement building had embraced the greatest struggle of my life. It seemed unfair to be just leaving, without some personal celebration to mark the milestone. It was quiet as we turned left from the driveway and drove up the hill.

I left behind some fears and demons, but also some hopes and dreams.

I was reflective as we drove home. Life had changed for me. Leaving Stan Cassidy gave me a final perspective: I would never, ever be the same. I had thought I would become an agile old fellow, bouncing grandchildren on my knee. I'd have a penchant for plaid flannel shirts and jeans. I'd be up early, doing odd jobs before breakfast. I'd still be canoeing, sailing, and doing manual labour into my seventies. I'd show my grandchildren how to hammer a nail. I'd take them on hikes into the woods. All gone.

I had to remind myself of what I had: Jill was beside me. *What more do I want?* I'd have to shift my focus, my ambitions in life. Still, I couldn't rally myself out of the doldrums. It should have been a happy day, a day I had been dreaming about for so long. Instead, I remained sullen as discouraging thoughts clouded my mood.

Reality set in as we drove up our driveway. This was our home. This was my life. I pivoted out of the car with Jill's help, realizing that this was only a new beginning. Life would be different, but that shouldn't exclude fun, laughter, and love.

Jill wheeled me onto the deck and around to the back door. When I opened the door, my face broke into a grin that I hope never fades — my children had decorated the kitchen with a hundred different-coloured balloons. It was magical. I was home.

CHAPTER 32
2000 TO 2002

Now that I was home, I had time to research the physical outcomes of brainstem stroke survivors. I suppose I was looking for some hope, but what I found, I didn't like.

Outcomes were varied: some people learned how to walk again, some stayed locked in, some returned to normal functioning with only minor deficits. Most survivors exhibited a variety of significant functional deficits after rehabilitation. But there seemed to be one constant: the functional gains attained by one year seemed to be the maximal rehabilitative state achieved. The improvements that were achieved after one year had little impact on the patient's overall function.

I proved that wrong — I attained useful function even after one year.

I started physical, occupational, and speech therapy, three times a week, as an outpatient at the Saint John Regional Hospital.

My new therapists had different approaches, with different results and different failures. I kept an open mind and attempted the variety of techniques they employed. Some physical therapists used a neurological developmental training (NDT) method while others used more traditional methods, and most used a combination.

I found NDT methods sometimes more effective, but not always so. Putting body weight on my affected right arm was supposed to decrease tone and then increase function, but it never worked for me. It did decrease my tone, but it didn't last long. That is not to say it wouldn't work for someone else.

I'm not delving any further into which methods helped me and which didn't — it would be too technical. Each therapist worked hard in trying to help me, and for that I am very grateful. I gained something from everyone.

It was not easy. It was hard to stay motivated when the exercises got monotonous with no or little reward. But looking back, it was well worth the time and effort.

Jill stretched my limbs four days a week, and a registered nursing assistant did so the other three days. I knew this might have to be a daily routine for the rest of my life, but my hope was that I could get by with less stretching in the future without sacrificing my well-being.

My speech was a pleasant surprise and represented the most significant functional improvement that occurred after the one-year mark. Two and a half years since the stroke, my speech was still improving. When I first came home, not many people could understand me, but now most could. I especially appreciated how I could be understood on the phone. I cannot emphasize how slow the progress was, but it happened.

I practised making my voice slide from low pitch to high pitch and vice versa, and singing. I also tried holding a note for as long as I could and counting out loud with complete pronunciation of each number. These exercises were boring (except for the singing), unrewarding (unless I looked back over time), but so necessary. I conceded that I would never have a natural voice, but my goal was to always be understood in normal settings.

Eating improved. I chewed with my front teeth because my tongue had a hard time moving food over to the side, but it was improving to the point that I was able to eat most anything as long as I was careful to keep my chin tucked in while swallowing — and no talking while I ate. I could drink anything, but I had to be very careful with clear fluids, sipping only small amounts at a time. When I forgot and looked up to see someone or something, I'd choke. I became so used to choking, I'd tell visitors, "Don't be alarmed if I choke. Please don't perform the Heimlich manoeuvre unless I turn blue." Thankfully, the Heimlich has never been needed, but I have been frightened by a few episodes of choking.

My body remained very stiff, refusing to turn or bend in any way. My balance was poor, but better. My left arm was quite functional — I typed the first edition of this book with it — but had trouble extending and reaching for things. My right arm remained stubborn; it wanted to stay close to my body with my elbow bent and my hand on my lap. My right hand was still contracted into a fist. It had improved for a while, allowing me to hold a utensil and eat with difficulty, but this never became practical. I tried writing with my right hand to promote increased function but struggled, fighting the tone all the time until I was exhausted and my arm would spring back to its preferred flexed position against my body.

I bought a power chair after I came home, or I should say my insurance company bought it for me on the recommendation of my occupational therapist. It took me a while to accept this into my life. My attempt at walking failed, as did using a manual chair — my right arm never became relaxed enough to reach down to push the wheel. While accepting a power chair was admitting defeat in one sense, it also gave me independence. I also realized that it didn't have to be a permanent defeat. I could still try to walk. I considered the chair a convenience; it was reality — a retreat, not a defeat.

The power chair, besides giving me much more independence, was comfortable. I remembered when I couldn't conceive of spending the rest of my days in a wheelchair and I wrestled with the feeling of being trapped; I had to get out. I still sat on a sofa for a change, but I much preferred my chair. It was more comfortable, and the irony was that I was actually trapped on the sofa.

My secret ambition was still to walk. I knew Mereille still held out hope for me, and my new therapists still took me for "walks," but I was a sad study in gait form. I didn't verbalize my desires too strenuously to my therapists; I didn't want the pressure. Every night, however, I prayed for the strength to continue.

Tara was often the only one home to help me. Colin and Beth helped when they were home from university, but mainly it was Tara. Every night, she would stand in front of my walker to prevent it from going forward too fast and also to help place my feet. Jill stood behind me, holding my right hand on the walker, steadying me, and pushing my legs forward as though I were stepping. We travelled from the kitchen to the living room, night after night.

I came home in April 2000 and we persevered for more than a year: night after night, the same unrewarding procedure. I feared my dream was just that — a dream never to be fulfilled. I would like to tell you that I said I was determined to succeed or I wouldn't give up, or some other noble, self-motivating statements, but it was fear that drove me, really.

I feared giving up. I feared failure.

I knew my obstacle to walking was rigidity. My hamstrings — the muscles behind my upper legs — and the muscles that pulled my legs together were too tight. If they could be relaxed, I might walk. My physiatrist told me about a new procedure that was becoming available: botulism toxin injections.

This neurotoxin is derived from the bacteria responsible for botulism, which produces a severe form of food poisoning. Botulism can result in death by paralysis. This neurotoxin, which causes the paralysis, is not harmful if injected into a targeted muscle; it does not spread throughout the body.

While the drug was going through the stages of being approved by the government, I had to keep trying to break the tone on my own. The more effort I put into lifting and bending my knee, the greater my tone became. Frustrated, hopeless at times, I kept banging into this wall of failure. The only path around that I could see lay in the medical procedure. This time, I couldn't back up and go around. I would have to wait. Meanwhile, I kept banging into that darn wall.

Jill was always behind me, emotionally and physically, my safety net. She wouldn't let me quit. It was physically challenging for her: holding my hand on the walker, checking my balance while pushing my feet ahead with her legs — an exhausting exercise. She never complained or took a night off, and in fact, she often had to remind me that it was time to walk.

Love had helped me get through the dark days and love still helped me, encouraging me to continue. Love was not only my safety net, but also the staff I leaned on.

Botulism toxin injections finally got approved for therapeutic use and my physiatrist gave me a small dose in September of 2000. It relieved the pain in my hamstring muscles and relaxed my legs, but at first this translated into little improvement in function. My arm and shoulder got injected in December, March, and June 2001. The partial paralysis from the toxin lasts about three months.

Sometime during this period, the tone in my legs imperceptibly reduced, and one day, to my surprise, I moved one foot a little past the other while I was practising with the walker. I'd like to report that I was soon walking, but as I had repeatedly learned in rehabilitation, there are no eureka moments.

June 2001. That dose did it! I moved one leg past the other — far ahead of the other. All by myself, without somebody pushing my leg forward. It started with one step, one leg, then the next time I took two steps, and after a few weeks, I was walking with only Jill holding my hand on the walker.

I was walking.

It was not pretty, nor was I independent, but it was a start. It had taken me more than two years, but my dream was fulfilled. Be ready to accept, but not without a good try. Sometimes progress is not possible, but there are always new breakthroughs in treatments and research.

Now that I was finally walking, I planned to get my right wrist stronger so that I could hold the walker by myself. Then I was going to learn to stand by myself. Finally, I'd be independent enough to stand, grab the walker, and walk to my destination. Then maybe quad canes instead of a walker; then maybe …

This would take years and a lot of work, but I had a plan, I had love to sustain me, and I had a dream to reach for. Never, ever, give up on your dreams.

CHAPTER 33
TWENTY YEARS AFTER: WALKING

The twentieth anniversary of my stroke was marked on May 13, 2019, which was around the time I was revising this second edition. I am now sixty-five years old. Jill and I live in a barrier-free home in Rothesay, New Brunswick, that we built fourteen years ago. I'm in a power wheelchair with left-handed controls, I can eat most anything with care, and I can talk well enough to be understood in a quiet environment.

The last twenty years have been a journey full of life's ups and downs. I finished the first edition (ending with the previous chapter) with the theme of finally achieving my goal of walking and the hope of independence in the future. Well, I'm not walking now, or even trying.

After I finished the first edition, I continued to walk with assistance as long as the botulism toxin was being injected into my legs. I was gaining distance; I progressed to walking from my back door to the driveway and back. I eventually could see that no matter how much I practised, it was doubtful I would ever be able to walk independently even with a walker because of my poor balance. I practised standing without assistance in front of a pole that I use to get into bed, with Jill by my side, but the longest time I could stand for was less than a minute. Balance control is a very complex system involving different body organs and pathways, and my stroke had affected the cerebellum and brainstem, two major control centres for this function. I tended to fall backward, and to prevent that I involuntarily thrusted my chest forward, putting strain on my lower back. I accepted that I would probably never walk independently, but walking was good for my heart, bones, muscles, joints, and lungs, so I kept it up.

I never achieved a good upright posture while walking; my chest was bent forward, with too much weight on the walker from my upper body. After I'd finish walking, my upper arms would be sore and weak from this weight. I did everything to relax the muscles so that my pelvis could come forward, but nothing helped. The spasticity forced my chest forward and my bottom back. Walking in a forward flexed position isn't an anatomically correct posture for the lower back to be in for such a long time, and it takes a lot of effort.

By 2008, my lower back had had enough, and I suffered a prolapsed lumbar disc that resulted in sciatic pain down my right leg. A disc is a gel-like structure covered by thick fibrous tissue that lies between the bones of the spine, and if they slip from that position, they can press on nerves leaving the spinal cord, causing severe pain along the length of the nerve. In the lower back, a disc prolapse impinges on the sciatic nerve, sending pain down a leg to the foot. The best cure is time. The disc will usually slide back into place with rest, but this can take weeks to months.

It took about a month for the pain to settle, and I spent most of that time in bed. When anything out of the ordinary happens to my body, the spasticity and tone of my muscles increases dramatically. If I'm anxious or upset about something, my spasticity increases and I end up with legs sticking out, arms unable to move my wheelchair control, and vocal cords unable to relax enough to speak. I would never be able to lie to Jill! My body knows when something is amiss before my brain does. If I'm catching a cold, I will get spastic the day before I have any recognizable symptoms. My body is aware of a viral attack before I am — how cool is that! So while I was suffering sciatica, my body was like a board and it took a lot of effort for Jill to get me up. It was better for Jill and my back if I remained in bed, but very boring. I listened to a lot of audiobooks.

However, even after I was free of pain, my body remained very tight. My muscle tone had reset itself to another level at rest, and even increasing the baclofen, the antispasmodic drug, above the maximum recommended dose did nothing to reduce the tone. I couldn't take a step with my walker.

After months of trying to give my rigidity time to relax on its own, my physiatrist decided I should be admitted to the Stan Cassidy Centre for Rehabilitation for assessment. I'm glad to report that since writing the first edition of *Locked In Locked Out*, the province of New Brunswick has built a new Stan Cassidy Centre for Rehabilitation, attached to the Dr. Everett Chalmers Regional Hospital in Fredericton. The new Stan Cassidy was fresh with the latest technology and assistive equipment for rehabilitation, and most importantly, the patients' rooms were so much larger than those in the old building. I was very pleased with the new centre, but not so much with myself. I was so tight the physiotherapist couldn't do much more than stretch me. After a week of this, I had gained nothing; I was wasting most of the day, so I told my physiatrist that I might as well go home. He assessed me himself and agreed, but decided that something further should be tried to decrease my tone.

He referred me to a neurosurgeon for an evaluation to see if I was a candidate for a baclofen pump. This is an electronic device that delivers the drug directly to the spinal cord, where ultimately the tone-reduction effect of the medication takes place. The pump is inserted under the skin of the abdomen and baclofen is delivered at a continuous rate via a catheter running under the skin from the pump to the spinal cord. The pump has to be refilled by needle every three to six months and the rate adjusted digitally by a handheld device. The advantage of this form of baclofen administration is that it bypasses the liver, where the drug can cause damage after long-term use, and much smaller doses of the drug have the same or better effect on spasticity than if taken orally.

After I was discharged from Stan Cassidy and had seen the neurosurgeon in Saint John, I was deemed an appropriate candidate and booked for a trial dose of baclofen to my spine. I was found to be tolerant of intrathecal baclofen (baclofen directly to the spine) and booked for surgery to implant the pump. While I was waiting for the surgical procedure, my muscle tone did finally relax; it was not as good as it had been before the disc prolapsed, but enough to allow me to start walking short distances.

I eagerly awaited implantation, because I secretly hoped for a big reduction in tone and possibly great advancement in my ability to walk. I knew the likelihood of this becoming reality was remote, but I couldn't help dreaming.

It was a fantasy, because I never got back to my pre–disc prolapse walking ability. It did improve my gait compared with before the surgery, but not before the prolapse. I reached a dose wall that I couldn't go beyond to reduce my tone because it would cause me to retain urine. This happened to me on oral baclofen, too, although only above maximum dose. I couldn't fully empty my bladder and experienced frustrating symptoms of frequency (wanting to urinate a lot), hesitancy (wanting to urinate but not being able to), and low abdominal pressure because my bladder was not emptying completely. It was difficult to sleep. This side effect of the drug was compounded by an aged, enlarged prostate and already abnormal bladder action due to my stroke.

However, I continued with the baclofen pump and had it replaced, which has to be done every five years, because it greatly reduced the resting tone in my legs. Now I didn't need them strapped onto my wheelchair when I travelled outside. Any rough terrain or bumps on a sidewalk caused the spasticity in my legs to increase, so before this, I'd had to keep my legs strapped to the chair or they'd extend straight out and slide my bottom out of the seat. It was painful to have my legs pushing against the straps when I rode outside in my wheelchair, and I loved getting out. With the baclofen pump, I could travel farther on rough terrain without using straps and enjoy the trip. The baclofen pump was well worth it for me, even if it didn't help walking.

Jill and I went back to walking, but it had become much more difficult: my forward flexion was worse, the distances travelled were much shorter, and the energy I expended was greater. Now, after a short walk, I was very short of breath and my heart raced, yet we continued. It became unsafe for just Jill and me to do this alone because sometimes my body would freeze in midtrip with nowhere to sit. In case I froze, we lined our route with chairs if we didn't have a third person to bring my wheelchair along behind us. Yet we continued. I feared giving up.

We continued walking with a walker in this fashion for a few more years until my lumbar disc prolapsed again one summer at the cottage. I spent most of a beautiful August on my side in bed, listening to audiobooks. This allowed me time to reflect on my attempts to walk. I was walking only to exercise my heart and keep my bones strong — I knew my dream of independent walking was over unless a medical breakthrough occurred. Was walking worth a possible long-term back problem? I decided my body was telling me to stop, and after talking this over with my physiatrist, we decided the risks of walking outweighed the benefits.

I haven't tried to walk in years. My heart may get lazy, my bones may get weak, but for now I'm comfortable and content. The average age of death for a male in Canada is now eighty and being in a wheelchair automatically reduces my chances of being average, so I would expect for me, seventy-five years would be more realistic. That's ten years from now, which slants my attitude toward maintaining my good health now, rather than risking an injury. My dream to walk has not come true, and I'm okay with that.

CHAPTER 34
TWENTY YEARS AFTER: OCCUPATION

I don't walk anymore, but I continue to exercise almost every morning. Jill stretches my limbs at least twice a week, followed by a shower. I'm independent in the shower; my right hand can hold and squeeze a bottle to pour shampoo onto my left hand. I use an arm bike, therapeutic arm bands, a motorized leg bike, and sessions of active limb muscle exercises. These activities are now for maintenance; I have no expectations that my function will improve.

I like to think of my day roughly like this: mornings are for my physical body with exercises; afternoons are for my mental fitness by engaging in committee work, online academic courses, and writing; and the evenings are for relaxing by watching TV, reading, or going to sporting events, movies, or the theatre.

When I accepted I wouldn't be able to work again after my accident, I became worried: what was I going to do with my time? I couldn't spend my afternoons watching TV — I'd go mad. Initially, writing *Locked In Locked Out* filled those afternoon hours, and I found the writing process very interesting but difficult physically and mentally. I type with one finger and had to learn a lot of rules about writing (which I obviously haven't mastered).

When I finished the book, I was lost. Now what? I wanted a hobby but I failed at everything I tried — most activities require two or, at the very least one, steady, fully mobile arm. My mind became obsessed with negative, guilty thoughts, I suppose because of the lack of occupation. The thoughts were so unrelenting and torturous, I knew I had to do something. *Shawnie boy, you are going bonkers! You're going off the deep end, old boy. You need something to keep your mind occupied.*

I started writing again. I don't think of myself as an author of published books; I decided I would write and enjoy the process without any expectations. It was similar to when I played the guitar. I must have written more than a hundred songs throughout my life and I enjoyed the process, but I never recorded or shared any of my work. It didn't matter; that wasn't my goal.

I have always been saddened by how children's personalities can be affected by events in life beyond their control. I personally experienced and witnessed this in my family medical practice. I decided to write a story based on this theme. I had a former professor of creative writing help me, and I read a few books on writing that proved to me I had a lot to learn.

My main character, Jacob, filled many hours and pushed those negative, obsessive thoughts from my mind. I thank him very much. I called the book *The Dove's Eye*, and because I couldn't be bothered to send the manuscript to publishers (at the time most didn't accept digital submission), I self-published it primarily for my family.

While writing *The Dove's Eye*, I decided to volunteer my time, so I became involved with local disability groups, which led to appointments to government committees: the Premier's Council on Disabilities and the New Brunswick Health Council. I have recently retired from the provincial boards after sixteen years but continue to be involved locally and on town committees.

Locked In Locked Out led to invitations to speak at many conferences over the years, locally and in the Maritimes, Winnipeg, Kingston, and Boston. This was very ironic because before my stroke, I would have been quite creative in inventing excuses to avoid public speaking. I really don't enjoy it, but I felt obligated to support my fellow stroke survivors in any way I could. I'm not speaking publicly anymore and have turned down a few invitations because I'm sixty-five years old now and officially a grumpy old man.

Dalhousie Medical School established a division in Saint John for New Brunswick medical students, and I was invited to direct an interprofessional program there. I did this for five years, and then for the next five, Jill and I were tutorial leaders for medical students in a course on professional competencies. All of these activities required a lot of preparatory reading, but I enjoyed interacting with medical students. I retired from these duties at the medical school this year.

I had time to pursue other interests after my accident. I've read hundreds of books, written three books (a historical novel, *A Forgivable Indecision*, was my third), and studied, through books and online courses, topics that interest me, especially spirituality, theology, and religious study on one hand and astronomy, cosmology, and astrophysics on the other. These seem rather diverse subjects, and I suppose what draws me to explore them is this question: how can I justify spirituality in an observable, measurable universe?

To try to answer this question — because my personal experiences, intuition, and comfort make me feel that God exists, or want him to — I engaged in a personal quest to explore God. I read the whole Bible over two years using a traditional guide to help explain its meaning, context at the time, and applicability for today. I read two books by well-known atheists. I took online courses about religion, spirituality, and the historical Jesus. I read books by spiritual thinkers; Bishop John Spong and the late Marcus Borg are my two favourite authors.

I am fascinated by the studies of astronomy, cosmology, and astrophysics. Space telescopes have yielded not only amazing visual pictures of our universe, but new data that improve our measurements and understandings.

I've learned a lot of scientific facts about the universe and scholarly opinions on religion, but to spare you, I will curb my enthusiasm and not discuss these matters here. The details of our universe are fascinating! All I will say is that after my personal quest, I have hope there is a place for God in our life.

When I say God, or Allah, I have no idea what that means: a deity, spirit, another dimension, or spirit world. I will never know, and I'm okay with that. My own experiences give me hope that God exists in some manner. I *knew* this stroke was about to happen, and I've experienced a few more events that some might say were coincidences, but I'm not so sure.

In summary, my personal exploration of spirituality in an observable, measurable universe is over and I'm satisfied with my conclusion at this time in my life. I have hope — I don't *know*, but I have great hope — that God *is* and an afterlife, dimension, or spirit world may *be*.

So eventually, I found things to fill my time. I had to actively seek out and explore activities to try, and then once I found them, other opportunities arose. I suggest to my fellow stroke survivors that if you're frustrated, bored, or feeling empty and can't resume past occupations, a good first foray into life after a stroke may be volunteering, if you're able, or joining a social group like a seniors' club. I am so grateful for finding a fulfilling life after being locked in.

CHAPTER 35
TWENTY YEARS AFTER:
LIFE

After my accident, we received disability income from insurance and are quite comfortable financially. Of course, I would have earned much more by working another twenty years.

When I reached the age of forty-five, I acknowledged that I should start slowing down. I was working eleven-hour days: to the hospital by 7:00 a.m. to see my patients, and then to my office by 9:00 a.m., where I saw patients all day, usually until after 6:00 p.m. It is always hard for a physician to slow down but still be available for patients. I had a plan. I was in the process of applying to become a preceptor, a doctor who supervises and teaches medical students or residents, in family medicine at Dalhousie Medical School. After a few years of being a preceptor, I would become more involved with the family medicine teaching unit at the Saint John Regional Hospital, which also might give me an opportunity to connect with a new graduate to take over some of my office hours. I would gradually work less and less, handing the rest of my hours over to a new doctor, until I could retire satisfied that my patients were being cared for. I had a plan, but as the saying goes, even the best-laid plans ...

A few years after I returned home, our little dog, Jenny, passed away at the age of eleven. We welcomed a new miniature German schnauzer, Maggie, to our life a year later. Maggie was a joy to have and passed away when she was twelve years old. We haven't had a dog since, and I miss that presence very much. Dog owners will know what I'm missing: the companionship and dogs' unique personalities and unconditional love.

My children are on their own, but they all live close by. Colin works as a project manager for an innovative health care company and is married to Sarah, a family physician. They have two children, Rebecca and Rachel. Beth became a speech language pathologist and works with autistic children. She is married to Brian, a musician, and they're expecting their first child. Tara was a palliative care nurse working in Ontario and then decided to become a doctor. She is now finishing her residency in family medicine here in New Brunswick.

If you remember, one of my first fears after I acknowledged I was locked in was that I wouldn't be able to play with my grandchildren. That fear proved to be only partially true. Becca and Rachel are special joys in our lives, as all grandparents would understand. They have accepted Grampy without judgment, as small children do, despite his wheelchair, clumsy arms, and weird voice. They often make sure I'm included by passing me toys, crayons, and food. I regret not being able to lift them up for a hug, hold their hand as we walk, or tuck them into bed, but those things can't be — and that's life. At least I'm here to experience the joy, to laugh and talk with them, to play chase and hide and seek (it is very difficult to hide in a wheelchair), and above all, to share love.

We spend three to four months each year at the cottage, a log cabin we call "On the Rocks." It is here, on the banks of the Saint John River where I spent the summers of my childhood, that I feel most at peace. My other immediate fear when I realized I was locked in was that I'd never be able to walk the rocks in front of my cottage. That fear was justified and prophetic, but as with my grandchildren, at least I'm here to enjoy the experience.

I admit, it is bittersweet at times. How I wish to be on the river in a boat or canoeing with my grandchildren or swimming in that refreshing water on a hot summer's day. When I start to feel bored or sorry for myself, all I have to think about are those who have never had the opportunity to experience these things and how fortunate I am to be here, watching ospreys and bald eagles soaring over the river, chickadees and squirrels vying for the seeds in our bird feeders, and boats sailing along the river.

When I've been bored, I have invented new things to do at the cottage, like photographing, identifying, and keeping a pictorial document of wildflowers. I've discovered an amazing variety of wildflowers along the dirt road of my summer community that cycle throughout the weeks of spring, summer, and fall. Next, I may try doing the same thing with insects. There is always something new to learn and do to fill our days.

Many things aren't the same anymore. I can't go down to the beach for a campfire in the evenings, so we compromise: my family brings the fire to me in our deck firepit. The joy of being together — telling stories, singing songs into the night, laughing — is still the same.

Some things have never changed. Jill is still beside me, and our relationship has deepened. I'm grateful for her love, daily care, and presence in my life. I would not have had the fight to emerge from being locked in or the ability to live my present life without her.

I am so grateful to be alive, and even more grateful not to be locked in. I'm reminded of this daily when I have a chat over tea with Jill or feel the sun, rain, and wind on my face or smell the pine on a journey down the cottage road. Being locked in twenty years ago has empowered me to become more aware and grateful for these simple pleasures of life.

I'm not happy this happened to me, but I'm not sad, either. I think I'm more tolerant, mellow, and self-reflective. I have learned and felt the value of love, and I appreciate the small, common elements of nature and living that we all tend to take for granted. It is peculiar that I must credit having been locked in for this grateful awareness of life.

Every day, I strive to celebrate each moment of good health and tranquility with joy and gratitude.

ACKNOWLEDGEMENTS

I wish to thank the folks at Dundurn Press for encouraging me to revise and update *Locked In Locked Out*. The original edition was published in 2002, and I had no intention of republishing the book until Dundurn Press unexpectedly expressed interest in the memoir early in 2019. I especially want to thank Rachel Spence, Dominic Farrell, and Elena Radic, editors at Dundurn Press, and Susan Fitzgerald.

I thank Randy Dickinson, present chairperson of the Premier's Council on Disabilities, past chairperson of the New Brunswick Human Rights Commission, and the founding executive director of the Premier's Council on the Status of Disabled Persons, for writing the foreword to the second edition of *Locked In Locked Out*. And thanks again to Stephen Willis for writing the foreword to the first edition.

I have to thank the people at the now defunct DreamCatcher Publishing, a small local company in Saint John, for publishing the first edition. At the time I wrote it, I had no aspirations of publishing my memoir, and I'm grateful they afforded me that opportunity. I especially thank my editor, Yvonne Wilson, and the late Elizabeth Margaris.

I thank all the people who offered me kind words about *Locked In Locked Out* and those who thanked me for sharing my thoughts and experiences since the memoir was first written. It was only the knowledge that I helped some people through loss that motivated me to rewrite and update a second edition.

Finally, I wish to thank my wife, Jill, for all the love and care. I would probably be in a long-term health care facility without her support. Not only did she give me the drive and support I needed to emerge from being locked in, she offered immense help as the first reader of this second edition. Thanks, Jill. Love you.